The Vitamin & Health Encyclopedia

The Vitamin & Health Encyclopedia

By

Jack Ritchason, N.D., Ph.D.

Woodland Publishing
Pleasant Grove, UT

While every effort is made to guarantee the timeliness and authenticity of all information researched and presented in this publication, the ever-changing nature of the many activities underlying the facts, figures, trends, and theories presented makes impossible unqualified reliance on the material herein. Further, nothing herein is to be construed as a substitute for consultation with a qualified expert. The author and publisher, neither directly nor indirectly dispense medical advice nor prescribe any remedies, and do not assume responsibility for those who choose to treat themselves.

Woodland Publishing, Inc.
PO Box 160
Pleasant Grove, UT 84062

Printed in the United States of America

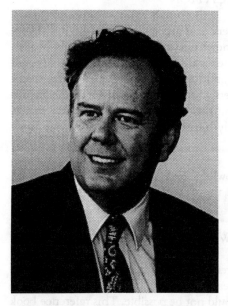

ABOUT

THE

AUTHOR

Dr. John (Jack) Ritchason has been in the health field since 1963 and has lectured nationally and internationally on herbs, vitamins, minerals, nutrition, and Iridology. He graduated in 1979, as a Naturopathic Doctor from the Arizona College of Naturopathic Medicine, a branch of the American University of Natural Therapeutics and Preventive Medicine.

He has his Ph.D. in Nutrition from Donsbach University and has done graduate work in Homeopathy in Missouri and also Florida Institute of Technology in Florida. Dr. Ritchason is a charter board member of Iridologists International. He is a member of the State Society of Homeopathic Physicians, is a Master Herbalist and (was the Dean of the Herbal Institute in Huntington Beach, California.)

Dr. Ritchason is a Life Member of the National Health Federation (NHF) and for a number of years held such positions as Vice President, Vice Chairman and Chairman.

Dr. Ritchason is a Registered Healthologist, Iridologist, Touch-for-Health Instructor and is certified in five different areas of Kinesiology. He has also completed his two year tutorial in Acupuncture. He is certified in both Colon Therapy and Reflexology. He has been involved as a teacher in all these sciences for 30 years. He is considered to be one of the top Iridologists and teachers of Iridology today. He is dedicated to the teaching of these principles. He has attempted to expand the knowledge to his fellow man to be able to help themselves and others. Since 1963, he has been sharing this knowledge with everyone who is willing to listen and the teaching aspect of it has been the most important part of his life.

DEDICATION

This book is dedicated to my very dear and loving wife who has always inspired me to continue seeking knowledge in all fields, especially health. It is my hope that this book will become a guideline to my posterity and others in their search for a better and healthier life. I am thankful that I have an all-just and merciful Heavenly Father who has given us the answer already for our physical problems on this earth. We simply need to search for the knowledge that is already here, for without health, we have nothing.

"I have been given a gift of knowledge from my Heavenly Father and if I do not share this with my fellow man, the gift will be taken away from me."

ACKNOWLEDGMENT

I wish to acknowledge some very good friends and colleagues of mine that without their dedication, tireless efforts, long hours, even into the wee hours of the morning, this book would not be possible. This reference book could not have become a reality without them. My sincere thanks needs to be extended to Linda Terrell and to her staff, Dr. James Terrell and their office manager, Mavis Roberts.

My prayer

It is my sincere hope and prayer that something i have said
would be beneficial to you—if not to you, your loved ones.
If i've done so then i've served you well.
I've also served my heavenly father well, Because he is my lord and master,
and because not only are you his children,you are also my brothers and sisters.
I thank him for the opportunity andI thank you for the opportunity.
May the good lord bless you with health and wealth,
If needed and may he keep you safe until we meet again.

God Bless You,
Sincerely Yours,

Jack Ritchason

God Gave us the laws of nature and
When we break those laws,
we pay for it here on this earth.

Table of Contents

Dr. Ritchason's
TEN GOLDEN RULES OF HEALTH

1. Stop putting poisons into the body.

2. It takes 5-7 times the normal amount of nutrition to rebuild and repair than it does to maintain.

3. Nothing heals in the human body in less than 3 months, then add one month for every year that you have been sick.

4. Have moderation in all things.

5. Make peace with nature.

6. Live closer to God.

7. You must take responsibility for yourself and your health.

8. Eat as much raw food as possible.

9. Exercise regularly the rest of your life.

10. Practice and learn to understand completely Hering's law of cure, which is "All cure starts from within out and from the head down and in reverse order as the symptoms have appeared."

Introduction

Life was intended to be rich and rewarding. Man was created and placed on earth to experience the full spectrum of life's opportunities. We have the capacity to know and enjoy the beauties of the natural world, the warmth of good interpersonal relationships, the fulfillment of achieving our goals. But central to our ability to enjoy life is the necessity of maintaining good health. The Apostle Paul understood this principle and it was written in John: "...1 wish above all things that thou mayst prosper and be in health..." (3 John: 2).

The Old Testament prophets were commanded to fast and to care for their bodies by using those natural foods available to them. Christ himself referred to his body as a temple (John 2:21) and followed the pattern of fasting and using wholesome foods to maintain it.

The same principles are true for modern man: We must sustain ourselves physically in order to be at our best intellectually, spiritually, and emotionally. The earth's abundance can still give us that sustenance, but our lives are now so complicated that we rarely can rely on diet alone to provide all the nutrients and chemicals our bodies require to function. Such commonplace and apparently harmless elements of daily living as refined sugars, white flour, daily stresses, and aspirin actually rob us of the nutrients we need to live! It is no wonder that vitamin and mineral supplements are so vital to our health: they restore the natural substances our bodies use up in keeping us going.

Today's health-conscious public is now realizing that natural vitamins, minerals, herbs and foods can also bring all-around better living. Athletes are finding that certain supplements give added strength and stamina. Vitamins, minerals, herbs and natural whole foods are helping thousands to control weight and keep in shape. As a beauty aid they are far surpassing any of the concoctions of today's cosmetologists. Students are finding that vitamins, minerals, herbs and natural foods enhance their alertness and mental capacity.

Good health comes from good food, from adequate exercise, and from giving special attention to particular areas of concern. With health as our goal and proper nutrition as our tool, we will find the peace without and within ourselves that the world seeks. This "Vitamin & Mineral Encyclopedia" is here to help achieve that peace, that balance, that whole life.

This book covers the different ways in how natural vitamins and foods can effect and balance our lives. This valuable information is meaningful, based upon how the reader views natural healing and the issue of how we as people, put our energy forth into the world. If we place our energy into situations which are unhealthy, in which the by-product of what we encounter is stress, then no amount of vitamins, minerals, herbs or natural foods will perform the miracle of right living from which well-being will result. Moderation in all things and knowledge about food and nature, will produce well-being. The important goal of life is in maintaining this balance which was given to us by our Creator. It is perfect and cannot be improved upon.

In medicine, we often encounter short cuts to health and well-being, by virtue that illness is treated as a condition without reference to the cause. This may be an over generalization, however, drug therapy is basically such. In many cases, we are discovering that some patients are ill as a result of iatrogenic (doctor-induced) and drug-induced illnesses. In alternative health, we too often see the same issue. People use vitamin and herbs because they are in a state of fatigue due to lifestyle issues and the hope is, that the vitamin and herbs will cure illness without a change in lifestyle. The truth is that these life supporting supplements can provide necessary elements needed by the body to heal and maintain a healthy life, but these vital substances do not heal unless there is a necessary change of living habits.

There is hope in being responsible as an individual and by using vitamins and herbs with proper food and food combining that the beauty of this creation can be recognized. The result is health and well-being in which one walks in peace and beauty!

So let us now approach health through gaining information that will allow us to meet our present health emergencies. Then depending on where we are health-wise, we can use this knowledge to improve our present health. Last, we can use this information to maintain ourselves and our families good health.

We must remember that drugs do not heal, they only change the form and location of the disease. In order to give vitamins and herbs a chance, one must allow the body to heal slowly. A permanent change of lifestyle is necessary to achieve health. It is imperative that you DO NOT STOP TOO SOON. Let the body finish its healing and rebuilding process. Proper food is very important. Unfortunately, some people think that all they have to do is take a few vitamins and everything will be all right. If they will not correct their choice of food that they are consuming every day and they will not get the proper exercise and rest, along with their thinking process of negativity and defeat, their problems will not stay away, they may not even heal.

You must stop putting poisons in your body. If you do not correct your choice of the foods you are consuming daily, your problems will come right back. Food can become our poisons, or it can become our medicine, and you can kill or cure from the kitchen table. The Creator has given us our right to choose that which we can have. Thus it is that we may choose a jelly doughnut brain, a pretzel spine, beer kidneys, coffee nerves, an alcohol liver, cigarette lungs, marijuana nervous system, a garbage dump colon, or anything else that we so choose. This includes all the side effects that go with it. We repeat to you, that you can kill or cure with your diet and your thinking and the most dangerous place can be the kitchen and the most dangerous instruments in the world can also be your knife, fork and spoon.

We trust you will gain individual health from the information that you receive, as you use this book. Remember, it is a study guide to healthful living. Use it well. Refer to this section occasionally to renew your goals. Just what is it that you want to achieve in life? Health? Wealth? A good relationship with your fellow man? Remember, we only pass this way once, we only have one body to live in, no place to buy spare parts, and I don't know where to turn it in for a new model. It is our hope that you will achieve the good health that can be achieved through learning the rules of health gathered in this volume.

God bless all of you!
Yours in good health,

Dr. Jack Ritchason

Preface

The Vitamin and Health Encyclopedia puts the information you need about supplements right into your hands. You don't need to wade through pages of meaningless detail to find what you want. It includes alphabetical listings of conditions which respond to vitamin and mineral treatment and of the characteristics and uses of individual vitamins and minerals as well. The information is basic, helpful and easy to find.

The first section lists many common conditions which may be treated with vitamins and minerals. Several suggestions are made for each condition: you may find that one vitamin or one combination works better than another for you. The second and third sections catalogue the vitamins and minerals themselves in alphabetical order, giving a little information about each one, listing the benefits of its use, and suggesting its best natural sources.

It is intended that you may use these sections as a cross-reference with the first if you wish. In the paragraphs explaining benefits you will find key words in italics to draw your attention immediately to the ailments or conditions concerned. This makes it easier and faster for you to find a complete list of optional answers to your particular question. For example, a quick glance at Section One will tell you vitamins C, D, and P might be helpful if you bruise easily. If you are interested in exactly how vitamin C affects bruises, simply look up vitamin C in Section Two and scan the page quickly until the word *bruises* catches your eye. Then you can immediately read exactly what you want to know about vitamin C without spending time looking through its other uses.

The fourth section gives you information on the Bach Flower Remedies (which are for the emotions in the body) which are actually low potency homeopathic remedies for such problems. Continuing in this section, you will find more information on homeopathic medicine and their uses.

Section five will fill you in on the building blocks of life. These are called amino acids. The body must have the proper abundance and the proper combinations at all times in order for the body to be healthy. Section six is about scientific advancements that include the following recent advancements that have been proven by their excellence, as follows: germanium, CoQ10, mercury toxicity and shark cartilage.

Section seven tells us of the raw glandulars. We can go back to Hippocratics, the father of medicine, who taught us the basis of using the heart for heart, liver for liver, and brain for brain, again following the principle of "like cures like." The remaining gems of information are information on Alzheimer's disease, candida albicans, multiple sclerosis and ALS. And we finish with one for the ladies, premenstrual syndrome.

Vitamins and minerals generally work to support and encourage the body's natural functions. Deficiencies of vitamins and minerals can cause those functions to slow down, to occur inappropriately, or to fail. For this reason, deficiencies must be corrected. Even those whose diets would supply all the vitamins and minerals they could normally use may have deficiencies for one reason or another. Stress at work, poor digestion, air pollution, pain, illness, even use of prescription drugs to combat disease can deplete vitamin and mineral supplies to deficiency levels. For this reason, regular supplements and a ready reference to symptoms and specific aids for problems as they arise can be your strongest ally in restoring and maintaining your health.

The beauty of vitamin and mineral treatment is that it is totally natural: it uses substances your body needs, substances your system was designed to use. Unlike treatment with drugs, vitamins and minerals add no foreign chemicals to the body and they produce no side effects. They do not take control of the body; rather, they maintain an environment in which the body regains and sustains control of itself. They can help ward off and prevent illness and disease from overcoming the body. Even in serious illness, they can give the body the fuel it needs to rebuild itself. Vitamins and minerals help the body correct minor and even serious health problems. They may not be able to correct inherited disorders. The body is the master; vitamins and minerals are the tools and materials for the body to rebuild itself.

VITAMINS AND MINERALS DURING PREGNANCY

The old saying "You're eating for two now" is pretty widely acknowledged as false. While a pregnant woman does not eat for two, her body does supply nutrients to her unborn child, providing it with the material to develop normally. The expectant mother's energy requirements may increase as much as 300 calories per day; a nursing mother can expend an extra 1,000 calories a day. Obviously, these are conditions under which the health of both mother and baby are dependent upon the mother's understanding of her increased need for nutrients. The pregnant or nursing woman should supply herself a good multiple vitamin and mineral supplement and be particularly aware of getting enough vitamins B, E, C, and D and sufficient calcium and iron. There were studies done in Europe that showed that a minimum of 400 IU of vitamin E is necessary to help prevent birth defects. There have also been studies done to show that women need a minimum of 1800 mg. total intake of calcium per day during pregnancy. This amount is even raised to 2400 mg. total intake during lactation to provide enough calcium for mother and child.

CHILDREN

Since vitamins and minerals effect the chemical reaction that changes food into useable proteins, carbohydrates and fats to build tissue and to supply energy, growing children need extra vitamins and minerals. They particularly require calcium, iron, vitamins C and B complex. Because kids expend so much energy and because they tend to supplement their diets themselves with sweets and junk foods, most of them get substantially fewer vitamins and minerals than they really need. In fact, sugar, sweets and carbonated drinks rob the body of calcium, B vitamins and vitamin C and other nutrients.

Ailments

ACNE

vitamin A/beta carotene, vitamin D, riboflavin (B2), niacin (B3), B complex, vitamin E and selenium, vitamin F, potassium, sulfur, vitamin C with bioflavonoids, chromium, zinc, pyridoxine (B6), black currant oil, acidophilus, EPA oils, pancreatin, pantothenic acid (B5), magnesium, flaxseed oil

ADRENAL GLANDS

pantothenic acid (B5), B complex, vitamin C with bioflavonoids, copper, zinc, chromium, L-tyrosine, enzymes, CoQ10, germanium, multiple vitamin/mineral, calcium and magnesium

AGING

vitamin A/beta carotene, vitamin D, vitamin (B13), pangamic acid (B15), B-complex, vitamin C with bioflavonoids, vitamin E and selenium, calcium and magnesium, potassium, sodium, enzymes, CoQ10, lecithin, multiple vitamin/mineral, Pycnogenol, germanium, glutathione, acidophilus, EFAs

ALCOHOLISM

B complex, particularly thiamine (Bl), pangamic acid (B15), folic acid, choline, potassium, zinc, pantothenic acid (B5), niacin (B3), vitamin C with bioflavonoids, calcium and magnesium, selenium, black currant oil, L-glutamine, vitamin E and selenium, EFAs, chromium

ALLERGIES

B complex, particularly pantothenic acid (B5), vitamin C with bioflavonoids, vitamin H, manganese, potassium, vitamin A/beta carotene, vitamin D, cyanocobalamin (B12), vitamin E and selenium, EFAs, calcium and magnesium, zinc, enzymes, hydrochloric acid (HCL), multiple vitamin/mineral supplement, manganese

ALZHEIMER'S DISEASE

Lecithin, vitamin E and selenium, vitamin C with bioflavonoids, B complex (Refer to Appendix, page 119) pyridoxine (B6), cyanocobalamin (B12), germanium, potassium, zinc, CoQ10, multiple vitamin/mineral, Pycnogenol, niacin (B3), L-glutamine, HCL and pancreatic enzymes, vitamin B1, L-carnitine, choline, iodine, zinc, manganese, B15, calcium and magnesium

AMENORRHEA

zinc, EFAs, vitamin E and selenium

AMNESIA

pyridoxine (B6), pangamic acid (BI5), B Complex, pantothenic acid (B5), L-glutamine, lecithin, niacin (B3), multiple vitamin/mineral

ANEMIA

B complex, particularly thiamine (Bl), pyridoxine (B6), cyanocobalamin (B12), folic acid, vitamin C with bioflavonoids, vitamin E and selenium, vitamin T, cobalt, copper, iron, molybdenum, pantothenic acid (B5), biotin, zinc, HCL

ANGINA

pangamic acid (B15), B complex, vitamin E and selenium, niacin (B3), CoQ10, lecithin, magnesium, potassium, EFAs, choline, inositol, vitamin C with bioflavonoids, copper, calcium and magnesium, L-carnitine, L-cysteine, L-methionine, omega-3 EPAs

APPETITE

thiamine (Bl), niacin (B3), cyanocobalamin (B12), B-complex, folic acid, vitamin C with bioflavonoids, vitamin H, zinc, vitamin A/beta carotene, calcium and magnesium, copper, multiple vitamin/mineral

ARTERIOSCLEROSIS/ATHEROSCLEROSIS

vitamin A/beta carotene, vitamin D, niacin (B3), B-complex, vitamin E and selenium, chromium, zinc, cystine, vitamin C with bioflavonoids, germanium, copper, multiple vitamin/mineral, EPA oils, lecithin, pyridoxine (B6), pangamic acid (B15), folic acid, iodine, vitamin H, EFAs

ARTHRITIS

B-complex, particularly pantothenic acid (B5), vitamin C with bioflavonoids, vitamin E and selenium, vitamin F, calcium and magnesium, phosphorus, sulfur, niacin (B3), pyridoxine (B6), cyanocobalamin (B12), folic acid, manganese, copper, germanium, silicon, sodium, potassium, L-histidine vitamin A/beta carotene, methionine

ASTHMA

cyanocobalamin (B12), pangamic acid (B15), B-complex, vitamin E and selenium, vitamin A/beta carotene, vitamin D, pantothenic acid (B5), pyridoxine (B6), vitamin C with bioflavonoids, calcium and magnesium, HCL, EFAs

ATTENTION DEFICIT DISORDER (ADD)

vitamin C with bioflavonoids, calcium and magnesium, pantothenic acid (B5), B-complex, vitamin E and selenium, niacin (B3), Pycnogenol, iodine

BAD BREATH

niacin (B3), pyridoxine (B6), B-complex, vitamin C with bioflavonoids, magnesium, enzymes, hydrochloric acid\HCL, zinc, acidophilus, vitamin A/beta carotene, vitamin E and selenium

BALDNESS/HAIR LOSS

B-complex, particularly niacin (B3), pantothenic acid (B5), pyridoxine (B6), folic acid, inositol, vitamin H, PABA, copper, vitamin C with bioflavonoids, vitamin E and selenium, zinc, iodine, chlorine, biotin, amino acid complex, silicon, tin, EFAs, HCL

BEE STINGS
thiamine (Bl), B-complex, pantothenic acid (B5), vitamin C with bioflavonoids, vitamin E and selenium, calcium

BELL'S PALSY
calcium and magnesium, B-complex, liquid mineral complex, cyanocobalamin (B12), vitamin A/beta carotene, vitamin D, vitamin C with bioflavonoids, lecithin, zinc, multiple vitamin/mineral, thymus glandular, homeopathic for virus, EFAs

BERIBERI
thiamine (Bl), B-complex, vitamin C with bioflavonoids, zinc

BIRTH DEFECTS
protein, B-complex, vitamin E and selenium, riboflavin (B2), folic acid

BLADDER INFECTIONS
pyridoxine (B6), inositol, choline, vitamin C with bioflavonoids, magnesium, potassium, acidophilus

BLEEDING (EXCESSIVE)
vitamin C with bioflavonoids, vitamin K, calcium and magnesium

BLOOD
to build-B-complex, pantothenic acid (B5), pyridoxine (B6), folic acid, cyanocobalamin (B12), vitamin C with bioflavonoids, vitamin D, cobalt, iron, to encourage clotting-vitamin K, to encourage coagulation-vitamin T, to dissolve blood clots-vitamin E and selenium, multiple vitamin/mineral, calcium and magnesium

BLOOD PRESSURE
to regulate blood pressure: niacin (B3), pyridoxine (B6), pangamic acid (B15), B-complex, vitamin E, calcium and magnesium, chromium, potassium, multiple vitamin/mineral, CoQ10, vitamin C and selenium, germanium, lecithin

BLOOD PRESSURE (HIGH)
calcium and magnesium, L-carnitine, potassium, vitamin E and selenium, zinc, CoQ10, EFAs, vitamin C with bioflavonoids, high fiber

BOILS/CARBUNCLES
vitamin A/beta carotene, vitamin D, vitamin C with bioflavonoids, vitamin E and selenium, germanium, iron, potassium, calcium and magnesium, iodine, zinc, B-complex, riboflavin (B2)

BONES
vitamin A/beta carotene, vitamin D, vitamin C , calcium and magnesium, fluorine, manganese, phosphorus, iodine, boron

BONES (FRACTURED)
vitamin A/beta carotene, vitamin D, vitamin C with bioflavonoids, vitamin E and selenium, calcium and magnesium, boron, iodine, HCL and pancreatic enzymes

BRAIN
inositol, potassium, sulfur, zinc, lecithin, niacin (B3), L-glutamine, vitamin E and selenium, Pycnogenol, germanium

BREAST CYSTS
vitamin A/beta carotene, vitamin D, vitamin E and selenium, COQ10, germanium, calcium and magnesium, black currant oil, iodine, EFAs

BRONCHITIS
vitamin A/beta carotene, vitamin D, vitamin C with bioflavonoids, vitamin E and selenium, multiple vitamin/mineral, zinc, calcium and magnesium, Pycnogenol, HCL, cysteine

BRUISES
vitamin C with bioflavonoids, vitamin K, calcium and magnesium,

Bach Flower Remedy #39, vitamin E and selenium, vitamin D, iron, pancreatic enzymes

BURNS

B-complex, vitamin C with bioflavonoids, vitamin E and selenium, PABA, zinc, Bach Flower Remedy #39, vitamin A/beta carotene, vitamin D, calcium and magnesium, germanium, Pycnogenol

BURSITIS

calcium and magnesium, vitamin A/beta carotene, HCL and pancreatic enzymes, vitamin C with bioflavonoids, vitamin E and selenium, cyanocobalamin (B12), germanium, zinc

CANCER

cyanocobalamin (B12), laetrile/amygdalin (B17), B-complex, vitamin C with bioflavonoids, vitamin A/beta carotene, vitamin D, vitamin E and selenium, germanium, calcium and magnesium, zinc, Pycnogenol, CoQ10, enzymes, shark cartilage, acidophilus, EFAs

CANDIDA ALBICANS

glandulars such as thymus, vitamin A/beta carotene, vitamin D, vitamin C with bioflavonoids, acidophilus, B-complex (from a yeast-free source). (See Candida Albicans in the Appendix, page 120), multiple vitamin/mineral, black currant oil, vitamin E and selenium, niacin (B3), iodine, L-Lysine, cyanocobalamin (B12), caprylic acid, pantothenic acid(B5), HCL, EFAs

CANKER SORES

niacin (B3), B-complex, folic acid, cyanocobalamin (B12), acidophilus, iron, L-lysine, zinc, HCL, vitamin C with bioflavonoids, vitamin A/beta carotene

CARPAL TUNNEL SYNDROME

potassium, pyridoxine (B6), vitamin A/beta carotene, vitamin D, vitamin C with bioflavonoids, calcium and magnesium, chromium, zinc, vitamin E and selenium

CHICKEN POX

vitamin C with bioflavonoids, vitamin E and selenium, vitamin A/beta carotene, vitamin D, potassium, zinc, calcium

CHOLESTEROL

niacin (B3), pyridoxine (B6), pangamic acid (B15), B-complex, choline, inositol, vitamin C with bioflavonoids, lecithin, vanadium, zinc, vitamin E and selenium, chromium, multiple vitamin/mineral, EPA oils, bulk/fiber, EFAs

CIRCULATORY SYSTEM

niacin (B3), pangamic acid (B15), B-complex, vitamin E and selenium, calcium and magnesium, oral chelation multiple vitamin/mineral, pyridoxine (B6), cyanocobalamine B12, vitamin C with bioflavonoids, lecithin, Pycnogenol, EFAs

COLDS

vitamin A/beta carotene, vitamin D, vitamin C with bioflavonoids, zinc, CoQ10, potassium, acidophilus, vitamin E and selenium, calcium and magnesium

COLD SORES

vitamin A/beta carotene, vitamin D, vitamin C with bioflavonoids, vitamin E an selenium, B-complex, acidophilus, calcium and magnesium, L-lysine, HCL

COLITIS

pyridoxine (B6), B-complex, vitamin E and selenium, vitamin K, calcium and magnesium, iron, potassium, acidophilus, vitamin A/beta carotene, vitamin D, chromium, zinc, cyanocobalamine (B12), multiple vitamin/mineral supplement, pancreatic enzymes, EFAs

CONGESTIVE HEART FAILURE
vitamin E and selenium, CoQ10, L-carnitine, potassium, calcium and magnesium, thiamine (B1)

CONSTIPATION
choline, vitamin C with bioflavonoids, vitamin E and selenium, magnesium, water, potassium, acidophilus, vitamin B-complex, vitamin A/beta carotene, vitamin D, bulk/fiber, EFAs, folic acid

CONVULSIONS
pyridoxine (B6), B-complex, calcium and magnesium, Bach Flower Remedy #39, vitamin E and selenium, pantothenic acid (B5), chromium

CUTS
pantothenic acid (B5), B-complex, vitamin C with bioflavonoids, vitamin E and selenium, calcium and magnesium, vitamin A/beta carotene, vitamin D

DANDRUFF
B-complex, iodine, vitamin E and selenium, pyridoxine (B6), zinc, calcium and magnesium, lecithin, vitamin A/beta carotene, vitamin D

DEPRESSION
cyanocobalamin (B12), B-complex, vitamin H, calcium and magnesium, flower essence, pyridoxine (B6), thiamine (B1), niacin (B3), choline, chromium, vanadium, zinc, lecithin, iodine, potassium, EFAs, vitamin C with bioflavonoids, L-tyrosine, inositol, folic acid

DIABETES
B-complex, vitamin E and selenium, chromium, manganese, potassium, zinc, silicon, vitamin A/beta carotene, vitamin D, calcium and magnesium, vanadium, multiple vitamin/mineral, EFAs,

cyanocobalamin (B12), lecithin, niacin (B3), acidophilus, L-carnitine, biotin

DIARRHEA

thiamine (Bl), niacin (B3), B-complex, folic acid, calcium and magnesium, potassium, acidophilus, silicon

DIGESTION

niacin (B3), inositol, chlorine, manganese, thiamine (Bl), riboflavin (B2), pantothenic acid (B5), pyridoxine (B6), cyanocobalamin (B12), B-complex, folic acid, sodium, zinc, HCL-pepsin, enzymes

DIZZINESS

pyridoxine (B6), pangamic acid (B15), niacin (B3), B-complex, vitamin E and selenium, choline, iron, multiple vitamin/mineral, lecithin, CoQ10, potassium, pantothenica acid (B5), vitamin C with bioflavonoids

DRUG WITHDRAWAL

B-complex, L-glutamine, pantothenic acid (B5), vitamin C with bioflavonoids, Pycnogenol, lecithin, chromium, vitamin E and selenium, calcium and magnesium, niacin (B3)

DRY SKIN

vitamin A/beta carotene, vitamin D, vitamin E and selenium, lecithin, EFAs, zinc, silicon

EAR INFECTIONS

vitamin A/beta carotene, vitamin D, vitamin B6, B-complex, vitamin C with bioflavonoids, vitamin E and selenium, manganese, zinc, acidophilus, manganese

EARS (RINGING)

manganese, multiple vitamin/mineral, zinc, calcium and magnesium, lecithin, vitamin C with bioflavonoids, vitamin E and selenium, B-complex, tin, EFAs, vitamin A/beta carotene, HCL and pancreatic enzymes

ECZEMA

vitamin A/beta carotene, vitamin D, B-complex, inositol, vitamin H, PABA, silicon, vitamin C with bioflavonoids, zinc, calcium and magnesium, HCL and pancreatic enzymes, folic acid, EFAs, vitamin E and selenium

EDEMA (SEE WATER RETENTION)

EMPHYSEMA

vitamin A/beta carotene, vitamin D, vitamin B15, vitamin B3, B-complex, vitamin C with bioflavonoids, vitamin E and selenium, calcium and magnesium, germanium, liquid mineral complex

ENDOMETRIOSIS

vitamin A/beta carotene, vitamin D, vitamin E and selenium, vitamin C with bioflavonoids, zinc, iodine, black currant oil, multiple vitamin/mineral, calcium and magnesium, iron, vitamin B-complex

ENERGY

B-complex, liquid minerals, pantothenic acid (B5), B12, iodine, vitamin E and selenium, vitamin C with bioflavonoids

EPILEPSY

vitamin B6, calcium and magnesium, folic acid, manganese, zinc, EFAs, choline, L-taurine and L-tyrosine, glycine, vitamin D, vitamin B-complex, chromium, niacin B3, acidophilus

EXHAUSTION/FATIGUE

vitamin B5, vitamin B12, vitamin B15, B-complex, folic acid, vitamin C with bioflavonoids, vitamin A/beta carotene, vitamin D, vitamin E and selenium, vitamin H, iron, manganese, zinc, potassium, iodine

EYE DISORDERS
vitamin A/beta carotene, vitamin D, vitamin B2, vitamin B12, B-complex, vitamin C with bioflavonoids, inositol, vitamin E and selenium, calcium and magnesium, zinc, niacin (B3)

FEVER
vitamin A/beta carotene, vitamin D, vitamin Bl, B-complex, vitamin C with bioflavonoids, sodium, water, enema, zinc, potassium

FOOD POISONING
folic acid, vitamin A/beta carotene, vitamin D, vitamin C with bioflavonoids, vitamin E and selenium, acidophilus, potassium, charcoal, zinc, EFAs, chromium, HCL and pancreatic enzymes, charcoal

FOOT PROBLEMS
vitamin Bl (for discomfort), iodine (for cold feet), vitamin B3, B-complex (for athlete's foot), acidophilus, zinc, vitamin A/beta carotene, vitamin D, vitamin C with bioflavonoids, L-Lysine, caprylic acid

GALLSTONES
vitamin A/beta carotene, vitamin D, vitamin B6, B-complex, vitamin E and selenium, calcium and magnesium, vitamin C with bioflavonoids, lecithin, choline, food enzymes, EFAs, fiber/bulk

GANGRENE
vitamin B15, B-complex, vitamin C with bioflavonoids, vitamin E and selenium, vitamin A/beta carotene, vitamin D, germanium, potassium, calcium and magnesium, zinc, germanium, Pycnogenol

GASTROINTESTINAL SYSTEM
vitamin A/beta carotene, vitamin D, vitamin B3, B-complex, vitamin B6, HCL-pepsin, food enzymes, zinc, sodium, B1, B2

GENITO-URINARY SYSTEM
vitamin A/beta carotene, vitamin D, B-complex, vitamin C with bioflavonoids, vitamin E and selenium, B6, sodium, potassium

GLANDS
vitamin A/beta carotene, vitamin D, vitamin C with bioflavonoids, B-complex, iodine, zinc, calcium and magnesium, potassium, (B5)

GLAUCOMA
vitamin A/beta carotene, vitamin D, B-complex, vitamin C with bioflavonoids, pantothenic acid (B5), magnesium, B6, B3, HCL, inositol, calcium and magnesium

GOITER
iodine, germanium, vitamin C with bioflavonoids, calcium and magnesium, B-complex

GOUT
folic acid, vitamin C with bioflavonoids, vitamin E and selenium, zinc, germanium, alanine, aspartic acid, glycine, bromelain

GROWTH
vitamin Bl, vitamin B2, vitamin B12, B-complex, chromium, iodine, iron, phosphorus, zinc, vitamin C with bioflavonoids, vitamin E and selenium, calcium and magnesium, protein/amino acids

GUMS/GINGIVITIS/PERIDONTAL DISEASE
CoQ10, vitamin C with bioflavonoids, vitamin A/beta carotene, vitamin D, iodine, iron, calcium and magnesium

HANDS
for numbness and cold hands: vitamin B6, B3, vitamin BI5, B-complex, vitamin E and selenium, iodine, iron, calcium and magnesium

HANGOVERS
vitamin Bl, vitamin B15, B-complex, vitamin C with bioflavonoids, calcium and magnesium

HAY FEVER
B-complex, pantothenic acid, vitamin C with bioflavonoids, potassium, vitamin A/beta carotene, vitamin D, vitamin E, germanium, zinc

HEADACHES
B-complex, particularly vitamin B3, vitamin B15, and choline, calcium and magnesium, vitamin C with bioflavonoids, pantothenic acid (B5), chromium, EFAs

HEART
Check for hiatus hernia, vitamin Bl, vitamin B15, B-complex, inositol, choline, vitamin A/beta carotene, vitamin E and selenium, vitamin K, calcium, and magnesium, phosphorus, potassium, vanadium, L-Carnitine, lecithin, EFAs

HEMOPHILIA
vitamin T, vitamin K, vitamin C with bioflavonoids, calcium and magnesium, vitamin B3, B-complex

HEMORRHOIDS
vitamin C with bioflavonoids, vitamin E and selenium, calcium and magnesium, lecithin, vitamin B6, vitamin A/beta carotene, vitamin D, choline, fiber/bulk, zinc, vitamin K, bromelain

HEPATITIS
lecithin, vitamin A/beta carotene, CoQ10, B-complex, Pycnogenol, vitamin C with bioflavonoids, vitamin E and selenium, vitamin B12, folic acid, germanium

HERPES
vitamin A/beta carotene, vitamin D, vitamin Bl, B-complex, vitamin C

with bioflavonoids, L-lysine, vitamin E and selenium, calcium and magnesium, lecithin, zinc, acidophilus

HYPERTENSION
B-complex, calcium and magnesium, B6, lecithin, iodine, vitamin C with bioflavonoids, fiber/bulk, EFAs, CoQ10

HYPERTHYROIDISM
vitamin A/beta carotene, vitamin Bl, B-complex, vitamin E, PABA, calcium and magnesium, iodine, vitamin B2, B1, B6, vitamin C with bioflavonoids, vitamin E and selenium, lecithin, EFAs, potassium

HYPOGLYCEMIA
vitamin B5, B-complex, vitamin C with bioflavonoids, vitamin E and selenium, calcium and magnesium, potassium, chromium, vitamin B1, B12, zinc, HCL and pancreatic enzymes, niacin B3, L-carnitine, L-cysteine, manganese

HYPOTHYROIDISM
iodine, B-complex, vitamin B2, B12, potassium, vitamin C with bioflavonoids

IMPETIGO
vitamin A/beta carotene, vitamin C with bioflavonoids, vitamin E and selenium, iodine, zinc

INFECTIONS
vitamin A/beta carotene, vitamin B5, vitamin B15, B-complex, vitamin C with bioflavonoids, iron, sulfur, water, vitamin E and selenium, zinc, germanium, iodine

INFERTILITY
vitamin E and selenium, zinc, vitamin A/beta carotene, vitamin B-complex, iodine, multiple vitamin/mineral, lecithin, calcium and magnesium, EFAs, zinc, germanium, vitamin C with bioflavonoids

INSOMNIA
vitamin B6, vitamin B15, B-complex, folic acid, choline, calcium and magnesium, iron, L-tryptophan, vitamin B3, liquid mineral complex, vitamin A/beta carotene, chromium, inositol

INTESTINES, LARGE
acidophilus, vitamin B6, vitamin E and selenium, calcium and magnesium, bulk/fiber, water

INTESTINES, SMALL
folic acid, inositol, calcium and magnesium, B-complex, pepsin

IRRITABILITY
vitamin B12, B-complex, calcium, manganese

JOINTS
vitamin C with bioflavonoids, sulfur, calcium and magnesium, sodium, silicon, manganese, copper

KIDNEYS
vitamin B6, B-complex, choline, vitamin C with bioflavonoids, phosphorus, calcium and magnesium

KIDNEY STONES
vitamin B6, B-complex, calcium and magnesium, vitamin C with bioflavonoids, vitamin A/beta carotene, vitamin K

LACTATION
vitamin Bl, vitamin B2, B-complex, folic acid, vitamin D, calcium and magnesium, vitamin A/beta carotene, multiple vitamin/mineral

LARYNGITIS
vitamin C with bioflavonoids, vitamin A/beta carotene, vitamin D, pantothenic acid (B5), iodine, zinc

LEG (CRAMPS)

vitamin Bl, vitamin B3, vitamin B6, vitamin B15, B-complex, vitamin E and selenium, vitamin H, calcium and magnesium, multiple vitamin/mineral, potassium, liquid mineral complex

LIVER

vitamin A/beta carotene, vitamin D, vitamin Bl, vitamin B6, vitamin B13, vitamin BI5, B-complex, inositol, choline, vitamin K, sulfur, lecithin, CoQ10, vitamin C with bioflavonoids, folic acid, EFAs

LUNGS

vitamin A/beta carotene, vitamin D, vitamin E and selenium, vitamin C with bioflavonoids, potassium, Pycnogenol, germanium

LUPUS

EFAs, vitamin E and selenium, liquid mineral complex

MANIC-DEPRESSIVE DISORDER

Amino acids: L-taurine, L-tyrosin, B-complex, liquid mineral complex, iodine, chromium, vanadium, B6, B2, B1, B12, vitamin C with bioflavonoids, calcium and magnesium, potassium, EFAs

MEASLES

vitamin A/beta carotene, vitamin D, vitamin C , vitamin E and selenium, calcium and magnesium, zinc, thymus glandular

MEMORY

multiple vitamin/mineral, CoQ10, germanium, vitamin E and selenium, lecithin, L-glutamine, amino acid complex chromium, B-complex

MENOPAUSE

B-complex, vitamin E and selenium, calcium and magnesium, lecithin, vitamin B6, B5, black currant oil, germanium, iodine, HCL and pancreatic enzymes, potassium,acidophilus, EFAs

MENSTRUATION
B-complex, particularly vitamin B6, vitamin K, vitamin E and selenium, calcium and magnesium, iron, zinc, iodine

MENTAL DISORIENTATION/ILLNESS
vitamin B3, B15, B-complex, calcium and magnesium, pantothenic acid B5, lecithin, Pycnogenol, flower essence, folic acid, vitamin H, B12, vitamin C with bioflavonoids, B6, iodine, vitamin E/selenium

METABOLISM
vitamin Bl, vitamin B2, vitamin B5, vitamin B6, vitamin B12, B-complex, folic acid, vitamin A/beta carotene, vitamin D, vitamin H, manganese, sodium, iodine, chromium

MIGRAINE HEADACHES
B-complex, particularly vitamin B3, calcium and magnesium, pantothetic acid B5, vitamin E and selenium, vitamin C with bioflavonoids, HCL and pancreatic enzymes

MISCARRIAGE (Prevention)
vitamin C with bioflavonoids, vitamin E and selenium, B-complex, calcium and magnesium

MITRAL VALVE PROBLEMS
calcium/magnesium, CoQ10, vitamin E/selenium, L-carnitine, EFAs

MONONUCLEOSIS
vitamin A/beta carotene, vitamin D, B-complex, large doses of vitamin C with bioflavonoids, potassium, vitamin E and selenium, germanium, acidophilus, thymus glandular, L-lysine, caprylic acid, zinc, HCL/pepsin, black currant oil, Pycnogenol, EFAs

MORNING SICKNESS
vitamin Bl, vitamin B6, B-complex, calcium and magnesium, multiple

vitamin/mineral, EFAs, vitamin C with bioflavonoids, vitamin D, vitamin A/beta carotene, vitamin E and selenium, vitamin K, iron, zinc

MOTION SICKNESS
vitamin Bl, vitamin B6, B-complex, magnesium

MUCOUS MEMBRANES
vitamin A/beta carotene, vitamin D, vitamin B2, B-complex, vitamin C with bioflavonoids, L-lysine

MULTIPLE SCLEROSIS AND ALS
vitamin B12, vitamin B13, B-complex, lecithin, vitamin E and selenium, calcium and magnesium, HCL/pepsin, liquid minerals (See Appendix for more detail, page 124), vitamin A/beta carotene, vitamin D, vitamin C with bioflavonoids, vitamin K, sulphur, acidophilus, potassium, multiple vitamin/mineral, germanium, caprylic acid, black currant oil, EFAs, pantothenic acid, CoQ10

MUSCLES
vitamin Bl, vitamin B6, B-complex, choline, vitamin C with bioflavonoids, vitamin E and selenium, vitamin H, calcium and magnesium, manganese, sodium, potassium, silicon, vitamin A/beta carotene, vitamin D, L-carnitine, liquid mineral complex, EFAs

MUSCULAR DYSTROPHY
inositol, vitamin E and selenium, B-complex, calcium and magnesium, L-carnitine, lecithin, silicon, potassium, multiple vitamin/mineral, EFAs

NAILS
vitamin A/beta carotene, vitamin D, vitamin B2, B-complex, iodine, sulfur, zinc, silicon, vitamin C with bioflavonoids, folic acid, calcium and magnesium, iron, (for white spots) zinc, EFAs, HCL and pancreatic enzymes

NEPHRITIS

vitamin B6, B-complex, vitamin C with bioflavonoids, vitamin E and selenium, calcium and magnesium

NERVOUS SYSTEM

vitamin A/beta carotene, vitamin D, vitamin Bl, vitamin B3, vitamin B6, vitamin B12, B-complex, choline, vitamin E and selenium, calcium and magnesium, manganese, sodium, lecithin, flower essense

NEURITIS

vitamin Bl, B-complex, lecithin, vitamin B12, calcium and magnesium

NICOTINE DEPENDENCY

vitamin B-complex, B12, calcium and magnesium, L-glutathione, vitamin C with bioflavonoids, vitamin A/beta carotene

NIGHT BLINDNESS

vitamin A/beta carotene, vitamin D, B-complex, vitamin B2 (twilight blindness), vitamin C with bioflavonoids, zinc, EFAs

NOSEBLEEDS

vitamin C with bioflavonoids, vitamin K, calcium and magnesium, vitamin E and selenium, B-complex, iron

NURSING

vitamin Bl, vitamin B2, B-complex, folic acid, vitamin D, calcium and magnesium, multiple vitamin/mineral, vitamin E and selenium, vitamin C with bioflavonoids

OSTEOMALACIA

vitamin A/beta carotene, vitamin D, calcium and magnesium, silicon, iodine

OSTEOPOROSIS

calcium and magnesium, enzymes/ hydrochloric acid, iodine, boron, phosphorus, liquid mineral complex, silicon, manganese, copper, sulfur, zinc, vitamin C with bioflavonoids, vitamin D, vitamin B6, vitamin K

PAIN
vitamin Bl, B-complex, folic acid, vitamin K, calcium and magnesium, vitamin C with bioflavonoids, Bach Flower Remedy #39, vitamin E and selenium, pantothenic acid B5

PARKINSON'S DISEASE
L-glutamic acid, liquid mineral complex, lecithin, enzymes/hydrochloric acid, calcium and magnesium, multiple vitamin/mineral, EFAs

PELLAGRA
vitamin B3, vitamin B6, vitamin B12, B2, B-complex, vitamin C with bioflavonoids, multiple vitamin/mineral

PERIDONTAL DISEASE
vitamin C with bioflavonoids, CoQ10, vitamin A/beta carotene, vitamin E and selenium, folic acid, copper, zinc

PHLEBITIS
vitamin C with bioflavonoids, vitamin E and selenium, lecithin, calcium and magnesium, B-complex, copper, EFAs

PINK EYE/CONJUNCTIVITIS
vitamin A/beta carotene & vitamin D, vitamin C with bioflavonoids, zinc

PNEUMONIA
vitamin A/beta carotene, vitamin D vitamin E and selenium, zinc, germanium, vitamin C with bioflavonoids, acidophilus, calcium and magnesium

POISON IVY
vitamin A/beta carotene, vitamin D, vitamin C with bioflavonoids, vitamin E and selenium, zinc

PREMENSTRUAL SYNDROME. (PMS)
vitamin E and selenium (800 to 1,200 IUs per day), vitamin C with bioflavonoids (3,000 mgs. per day), pituitary and thyroid glandulars, black currant oil, potassium, iodine, B-complex, pantothenic acid B5, calcium and magnesium, vitamin B6, EFAs, zinc, iron, chromium, vitamin A/beta carotene, acidophilus. (See Premenstrual Syndrome in the Appendix, page 126. Also refer to Candida Albicans.)

PROSTATE DISORDERS
vitamin E and selenium, vitamin F, zinc, vitamin A/beta carotene, vitamin D, lecithin, calcium and magnesium, Pycnogenol, acidophilus, EFAs, fiber/bulk, amino acids (glycine, alanine and glutamic acid), vitamin B6

PSORIASIS
vitamin A/beta carotene, vitamin D, inositol, vitamin C with bioflavonoids, vitamin E and selenium, vitamin B-complex, zinc, lecithin, calcium and magnesium, Pycnogenol, folic acid, shark cartilage, EFAs, copper, HCL/pancreatic enzymes, vitamin B12, silicon

RAYNAUD'S DISEASE
calcium and magnesium, vitamin E and selenium, EFAs, niacin (B3)

REPRODUCTIVE SYSTEM
vitamin A/beta carotene, vitamin D, vitamin B2, B-complex, vitamin E and selenium, manganese, zinc, iodine, lecithin, calcium and magnesium

RESPIRATORY SYSTEM
vitamin A/beta carotene, vitamin D, vitamin E and selenium, vitamin C with bioflavonoids, zinc, Pycnogenol

RESTLESSNESS
vitamin B3, vitamin B6, B-complex, calcium and magnesium, multiple vitamin/mineral, silicon

RHEUMATIC FEVER
vitamin A/beta carotene, B-complex, vitamin C with bioflavonoids, vitamin E and selenium, PABA, CoQ10, acidophilus, calcium and magnesium, germanium

RHEUMATISM
vitamin B15, B-complex, vitamin P, calcium and magnesium, sodium, B6, HCL/pepsin, reduce protein intake, histidine, EFAs, vitamin E and selenium, copper, shark cartilage

RICKETS (See Osteomalcia)

SCHIZOPHRENIA
germanium, niacin B3, B-complex, check for hypoglycemia and hypothyroidism, calcium and magnesium, iodine, EFAs, chromium and vanadium, B1, B5, B6, choline

SCIATICA NERVE
B-complex, lecithin, calcium and magnesium, silicon, homeopathic remedy, liquid mineral complex

SCURVY
vitamin A/beta carotene, vitamin D, vitamin Bl, vitamin B3, B-complex, vitamin C with bioflavonoids

SHINGLES
vitamin B12, B-complex, calcium and magnesium, L-Lysine, vitamin C with bioflavonoids, vitamin E and selenium, zinc, Bach Flower Remedy # 39

SHOCK
vitamin B5, B-complex, vitamin C with bioflavonoids, Bach Flower Remedy #39, B3, vitamin E and selenium

SINUSITIS
vitamin A/beta carotene, vitamin B5, B-complex, vitamin C with bioflavonoids, vitamin E and selenium, zinc, homeopathic remedy, CoQ10

SKIN CANCER
CoQ10, black currant oil, vitamin A/beta carotene, vitamin D, zinc, vitamin C with bioflavonoids, vitamin E and selenium, EFAs

SKIN DISORDERS
vitamin A/beta carotene, vitamin D, vitamin B2, vitamin B3, vitamin B6, B-complex, vitamin E and selenium, folic acid, vitamin F, vitamin H, PABA, iodine, iron, sulfur, silicon, zinc, black currant oil, lecithin, B12, B5, EFAs, vitamin C with bioflavonoids

SNAKEBITE
vitamin A/beta carotene, vitamin D, vitamin C with bioflavonoids, vitamin K, calcium and magnesium, B5, HCL/pepsin

SORES
vitamin A/beta carotene, vitamin D, vitamin B2, vitamin B3, B-complex, vitamin C with bioflavonoids, vitamin E and selenium, folic acid, zinc, EFAs

SORE THROAT
vitamin A/beta carotene, vitamin D, vitamin B2, vitamin C with bioflavonoids, iodine, acidophilus, zinc

STAPH INFECTIONS
vitamin C with bioflavonoids, vitamin A/beta carotene, vitamin D, acidophilus, zinc, iodine

STRESS (Mental and Physical)
B-complex, particularly vitamin B2, vitamin B5, vitamin B6, vitamin B15, folic acid, vitamin C with bioflavonoids, vitamin E and selenium, PABA, calcium and magnesium, phosphorus, Bach Flower Remedy #39, lecithin, zinc, potassium, L-tyrosine

STROKE
B-complex, large doses of vitamin B6, vitamin C with bioflavonoids, calcium and magnesium, #39 Bach Flower Remedy, EFAs, vitamin A/beta carotene, vitamin E and selenium, potassium, liquid mineral complex, lecithin, CoQ10, germanium

SUNBURN/SUNSTROKE
B-complex, vitamin C with bioflavonoids, PABA, potassium, vitamin K, vitamin E and selenium, sodium

SYPHILIS
B-complex, vitamin C with bioflavonoids, germanium, acidophilus, zinc

TACHYCARDIA (Rapid Heart Beat)
magnesium, potassium, B1, B3, selenium

TASTE
zinc, B-complex

TEETH
vitamin A/beta carotene, vitamin D, vitamin B3, vitamin B5, vitamin B6, B-complex, vitamin C with bioflavonoids, calcium and magnesium, chlorine, fluorine, iodine, phosphorus

THROMBOSIS

vitamin E and selenium, vitamin C with bioflavonoids, calcium and magnesium, B3

TUMORS (Fatty)

lecithin, CoQ10, germanium, vitamin A/beta carotene, vitamin D

ULCERS

vitamin A/beta carotene, vitamin D, B-complex, folic acid, vitamin C with bioflavonoids, vitamin E and selenium, vitamin U, calcium and magnesium, vitamin B6, vitamin K, zinc, HCL or enzymes, L-glutamine, potassium

VARICOSE VEINS

vitamin C with bioflavonoids, vitamin E and selenium, calcium, and magnesium, lecithin, potassium, vitamin A/beta carotene, vitamin D, zinc, copper, vitamin K, bromelain, L-lysine

VENEREAL DISEASE

vitamin A/beta carotene, vitamin D, vitamin C with bioflavonoids, zinc, vitamin E and selenium

VIRAL INFECTIONS

vitamin A/beta carotene, vitamin D, vitamin C with bioflavonoids, L-lysine, zinc, black currant oil, homeopathic remedy, EFAs

VISION

vitamin A/beta carotene, vitamin D, vitamin B2, vitamin B3, B-complex, vitamin C with bioflavonoids, vitamin E and selenium

WARTS

vitamin A/beta carotene, vitamin D, vitamin E and selenium, silicon, vitamin B-complex, vitamin C with bioflavonoids, zinc, black currant oil, L-cysteine, EFAs

WATER RETENTION/EDEMA
vitamin B6, vitamin C with bioflavonoids, CoQ10, vitamin E and selenium, potassium

WEAKNESS (General)
vitamin Bl, vitamin B6, B-complex, vitamin C with bioflavonoids, vitamin E and selenium, potassium, B12, iodine

WEIGHT LOSS
vitamin Bl, vitamin B6, B-complex, inositol, choline, calcium and magnesium, L-phenylalanine, vitamin C with bioflavonoids, vitamin E and selenium, iodine, L-carnitine, food enzymes, chromium, fiber/bulk, EFAs

WOUNDS
vitamin A/beta carotene, vitamin D, vitamin B5, B-complex, vitamin C with bioflavonoids, vitamin E and selenium, zinc

Vitamins

Vitamins are organic substances necessary for life. We have to ingest vitamins in or with our food. As a matter of fact, the body cannot use vitamins without minerals. The food we eat is composed of proteins, carbohydrates, and fats which the body converts into energy in a form it can use. In order to do that, the body must have the proper amounts and kinds of vitamins. Balanced vitamins act like a catalyst for use of other nutrients; they are not themselves used, but they start and maintain the chemical reaction through which you burn calories and use up the fuel that feeds your body.

Most vitamins are water soluble. That is, they combine with water in the body to do their job, and then they are carried off and excreted in the urine. Most vitamins remain in your system for two-to-three hours at the longest before they are eliminated. In order to assure day-long vitamin levels, water-soluble vitamins must be taken regularly—either by eating a proper diet or by taking supplemental vitamins such as found in tablet or capsule form.

The oil-soluble vitamin, A, D, and E, are needed for fat assimilation. If for some reason your diet does not include sufficient fat, the oil-soluble vitamins are available in "dry" or water-soluble form. In any case, vitamins should be taken before—not between and not in place of meals. Ideally, they should be taken with breakfast, with lunch, and with dinner, but if your schedule allows you only one time a day for vitamins, make that time with breakfast and try to use time release vitamins. Feed your body every five hours for maximum efficiency.

HOW VITAMINS FUNCTION BEST

Try to balance your vitamins to work together. The B-complex, for example, is a group of twenty-two similar vitamins. Even though they are all distinct, none of them work as well alone as the entire group does together. They are never found singly in nature; they are always all there. Other vitamins have partners as well; it is a good idea to combine them for effectiveness.

Vitamin A functions best with B-complex, vitamin D, vitamin E, calcium, phosphorus, and zinc.

Vitamin D functions best with vitamin A, vitamin C, choline, calcium, and phosphorus.

Vitamin E functions best with B-complex, inositol, vitamin C, manganese and selenium.

Vitamin C (ascorbic acid) functions best with bioflavonoids, calcium, and magnesium.

Folic acid (folacin) functions best with B-complex and vitamin C.

Niacin functions best with vitamin B1, vitamin B2, B-complex and vitamin C.

Vitamin B1 (thiamine) functions best with B-complex, vitamin B2, folic acid, niacin, vitamin C, and vitamin E.

Vitamin B2 (riboflavin) functions best with vitamin B6, B-complex, vitamin C, and niacin.

Vitamin B6 (pyridoxine) functions best with vitamin B1, vitamin B2, B-complex, pantothenic acid, vitamin C, and magnesium.

Vitamin B12 (cyanocobalamin) functions best with vitamin B6, B-complex, vitamin C, folic acid, choline, inositol, and potassium.

Calcium functions best with vitamin A, vitamin C, vitamin D, iron, magnesium, and phosphorus.

Phosphorus functions best with calcium, vitamin A, vitamin D, iron, and manganese.

Iron functions best with vitamin B12, folic acid, vitamin C, and calcium.

Magnesium functions best with vitamin B6, vitamin C, vitamin D, calcium, and phosphorus.

Zinc functions best with vitamin A, calcium, and phosphorus.

TOXIC EFFECTS OF VITAMINS

A few vitamins may have toxic effects if taken in massive doses over a long period of time. Watch massive intake of vitamins A and D; avoid combining vitamin A with mineral oil or vitamin E with inorganic iron. Typically synthetic vitamins cause reactions. Natural vitamins, even in high doses, are reasonably safe if used wisely.

VITAMIN A

Because vitamin A is fat soluble, it requires fats as well as minerals for proper absorption in the digestive tract. The body can store vitamin A. As a matter of fact, very large daily doses of vitamin A over a period of months can produce toxic effects. The average dosage of vitamin A is 25,000 to 100,000 units depending on body stresses.

Vitamin A occurs in two forms—performed vitamin A, called retinol (found only in foods of animal origin), and provitamin A, known as beta-carotene (provided by foods of both plant and animal origin).

How much "A" is too much? According to Dr. Ray Yancey, research has showed the following: *"University of Pennsylvania, School of Medicine and The Simon Greenberg Foundation* states: "We constantly receive inquiries regarding vitamin A—whether or not it is toxic . . . 40,000 I.U. . . . is the same amount of vitamin A you would receive if you ate a three ounce portion of calf's liver in a restaurant." Pretty dangerous, huh? But maybe that analogy isn't scientific enough for you—so consider the following:

The University of Pennsylvania, School of Medicine, Department of Dermatology: "In the treatment of acne vulgaris, the use of vitamin A was highly efficacious in doses of 300,000 units for women and 400,000 to 500,000 units for men. The danger of hypervitaminosis A in this dosage range has been exaggerated. Vitamin A is a valuable drug for treating stubborn, severely inflammatory acne vulgaris."

Ostwald & Briggs: "The review of Nieman and Obnbink indicates that, for adults, 1 million I.U. is a toxic dose. Chronic toxic dose for children 1 to 3 years of age was calculated to be about 100,000 I.U per day with a six month period required before toxicity occurs. It has been reported that cortisone decreases the tolerance to vitamin A and moderate amounts of vitamin E or K renders excess amounts of vitamin A harmless."

International Journal of Vitamin and Nutrition Research: "It was determined that a three and one-half year intake of 375,000 I.U. per day for a 150 lb. adult is necessary before any symptoms of vitamin A toxicity appear. "

Studies have shown that vitamin A lowers the incidence of lung cancer and also that it may prove valuable for people who don't smoke, too. Vitamin A may also protect against the "secondhand" cigarette smoke that is inadvertently inhaled by nonsmokers.

Benefits

In general, vitamin A serves to maintain the body's thin coverings and also it mucous membranes in various organs, systems, and glands. Specifically, vitamin A:

- counteracts night blindness and heals disorders of the eyes
- helps treat such skin problems as acne, impetigo, psoriasis, boils, carbuncles, and open ulcers when applied directly
- builds resistance to colds and to infections, particularly in the gastrointestinal, urinary, and respiratory systems
- promotes healing of broken bones and damaged skin or organs
- aids in treatment of emphysema and hyperthyroidism
- promotes healthy bones, skin, hair, teeth and gums
- maintains balance of sex hormones
- shortens the duration of diseases
- cancer

Natural Sources

Green and yellow vegetables, eggs, milk and dairy products, margarine, yellow fruits, liver, fish liver oil, lemon grass

Deficiencies

Loss of smell, birth defects, fatigue, growth, acne, dry hair, growth retardation, infections, night blindness, hyperketosis, infertility, insomnia, weight loss, dry skin, dry mouth, thickened scaly skin on the palms and soles of the feet

BETA-CAROTENE (Provitamin A carotenoid)

Beta-carotene is the yellowish pigmented substance that colors yellow, orange or dark green vegetables and is converted in the body into vitamin A. In 1928, the research of Dr. B. Von Euler revealed that beta-carotene was the source or provitamin for vitamin A. Beta-carotene is part of a family of related vital food substances named carotenoids.

Beta-carotene must be converted in the body to vitamin A. One molecule of beta-carotene can be converted by the body to two molecules of vitamin A. This is done by a special enzyme produced by the body and present in the intestines where it does much of its work.

This conversion process is in one direction only: One molecule of beta-carotene can be converted into two molecules of vitamin A, but vitamin A cannot be reconstructed back into beta-carotene. Beta-carotene in the diet is one of the main nontoxic suppliers of vitamin A and by a special ability of the body can yield only the necessary amount as it is needed.

Your body can change the 50 or more of the carotenoids thus far identified, into vitamin A. Conversion to vitamin A first must take place before the carotenoids can be used by or stored in the liver. Enzymes in the intestines divide the one beta-carotene molecule, into two molecules of vitamin A, before it is absorbed into the bloodstream through the intestinal wall. This allows for rapid utilization of the converted vitamin A. However not all, or even a majority of the carotene is converted to vitamin A. A large portion of the beta-carotene enters the circulation and tissues intact to be utilized as carotene as necessary as is vitamin A to the functions of the body systems.

Beta-carotene is not toxic in any known amounts. Should a slight discoloration of the skin occur after taking amounts of carrot juice, there is no need for alarm as this will soon disappear. This discoloration should be a welcome sign as it is evidence that the toxins or impurities which have been clogging up the liver, are being dissolved. Often these impurities are released in such quantities that the intestinal and urinary organs are unable to cope with the overflow and they are then passed into the lymph for discharge through the pores of the skin. So you have clear proof that the carrot juice is doing its valuable work. Due to its cleansing and nutritious abilities, large constantly supplied amounts of beta carotene tend to cleanse the liver by way of dumping the contents of the gall bladder emptying bile rapidly into the system, a condition often misdiagnosed as yellow jaundice, but generally harmless.

Beta-carotene is superior to vitamin A in wound healing, speeding up the healing effect. Beta-carotene is a powerful antioxidant and known for its ability to promote the healing of other diseases including cancer. Beta-carotene is gaining a reputation as being a strong anti-cancer agent. Many researchers are now saying that people who have a high beta-carotene intake may have a lower risk of cancer. It averts many chemical reactions in the body that are often linked to cancer development. Carrot juice is especially rich in beta-carotene.

Beta-carotene helps to protect the mucous membranes of the mouth, lungs, throat and nose. It also helps protect vitamin C from oxidation, which allows your vitamin C to work better.

Like vitamin A itself, beta-carotene is fat-soluble and fat storable. The body decreases the conversion of beta-carotene to vitamin A when blood levels of vitamin A are high. This is due to the body manufacturing of a special beta-carotene splitting enzyme that is the chief agent used by the body to split the carotene into two vitamin A's. In the case of a saturated amount of vitamin A, being present in the body, the manufacturing of this enzyme is retarded, thus preventing the over supply of vitamin A.

Natural Sources

Yellow and orange vegetables (carrots, sweet potatoes and pumpkins), green leafy vegetables (spinach, broccoli, collard greens, turnip greens and peppers), and yellow and orange fruits (papayas, oranges, apricots, peaches and cantaloupes)

Deficiencies

Atherosclerosis, breast cancer, cataracts, cervical dysplasia, colorectal cancer, hives, lung cancer, ovarian cancer, PMS, prostate cancer, psoriasis

ACIDOPHILUS

Acidophilus is a friendly bacteria in the bowel. The flora in the bowel can determine the state of health in an individual. Acidophilus protects your colon from cancer. It is normally established at birth. You need proper amounts of acidophilus in order to aid digestion and assimilation of foods. The first acidophilus introduced in a baby is through the colostrum from the mother's milk.

Acidophilus protects us from E. coli, which causes cancer to form in the colon. Acidophilus is lost through the taking of antibiotics, *excessive* flushing of the colon through enemas or colonics; excessive intake of red meats which have antibiotics in them; coffee also destroys it. Antihistamines, penicillin, and sulpha drugs all destroy the friendly bacteria in the bowel. Cortisone and prednisone also destroy aciophilus in the colon. Birth control pills also destroy acidophilus.

Putrification is caused by unfriendly bacteria, and acid foods prevent putrification for many of the unfriendly bacteria cannot live in acid medium. The acidophilus bacillus has the power of fixing itself to the wall of the stomach and exerting its good influence on the contents of the stomach. What this means is the intestines are kept free for longer periods of time from harmful bacteria. We manufacture our own B-12 if we have adequate amounts of acidophilus in the bowel.

Such people as Illya Metchnikoff, professor at the Pasteur Institute in Paris, has advanced the theory that unfriendly microbes in the intestine may be responsible for premature death and disease. He believes that the intake of acidophilus can give us a long and healthy life. He says the main therapeutical effect of acidophilus lies in its ability to reduce putrification. It needs to be stressed that taking acidophilus will in no way harm the effectiveness of antibiotics. Anyone taking any kind of antibiotic for any length of time should supplement his diet with acidophilus.

To finalize, Metchnikoff felt that a man consuming acidophilus every day of his life should be able to live to 150 years of age. Disease will use up the friendly flora also. The bowel should be acid and cidophilus provides this. The ratio of bacteria in the bowel should be at least 80 percent acidophilus to 20 percent of the unfriendly bacteria. This has been found to be reversed in unhealthy people.

The Pasteur Institute in Paris, France says that man dies of one disease and it is called autointoxication (reabsorption of the poisons back into the bloodstream that the body is attempting to eliminate). Thus, we drown in our own poisonous wastes which weakens our immune system to such a point that our weakest link in our chain takes us out. Then the doctor will put on our death certificate that we died of tuberculosis, cancer and so forth.

VITAMIN B1 (Thiamine)

Vitamin B1 is necessary for the body to make full use of its carbohydrate intake. Sometimes called the "morale vitamin," B1 strengthens the nervous system and can improve mental attitude. It helps all kinds of stress, so the need for this vitamin increases during illness, trauma, anxiety, and postsurgical periods.

Women who are pregnant, nursing, or taking birth control pills have increased needs for vitamin B1, as do smokers, drinkers, and those who consume a great deal of sugar or caffeine.

Vitamin B1 is water soluble and must be replaced daily.

Benefits

- necessary in treatment of beriberi, neuritis, and alcoholism
- aids digestion, particularly of carbohydrates
- helps fight air- or seasickness
- maintains functioning of the nervous system, muscles, heart

- aids in treatment of herpes zoster (shingles)
- helps relieve dental postoperative pain
- promotes growth
- improves mental attitude
- repels biting insects
- helps regulate the heart

Natural sources

Whole wheat, oatmeal, peanuts, bran, most vegetables, dairy products, rice husks, dried yeast, brewer's yeast and blackstrap molasses

Deficiencies

Anorexia, senility, confusion, constipation, coordination impairment, depression, labored breathing (dyspnea), GI upset, edema, fatigue, irritability, memory loss, muscle atrophy, nervousness, numbness hands and feet, pain hypersesitivity, palpitations, weakness, heart irregularity

VITAMIN B2 (Riboflavin)

Vitamin B2 helps the body digest fats, proteins, and carbohydrates and convert them into energy it can use. Riboflavin is also essential for the production of red blood cells, and antibodies. When used with vitamin A, riboflavin helps to maintain mucous membranes in the digestive tract. This vitamin is necessary for cell respiration and growth, and facilitates the use of oxygen by body tissues. This vitamin is required for any tissue repair such as burns or other injuries, and plays a vital role during conditions of physical stress such as surgery, fevers, and alcoholism. Animal studies have shown a correlation between the formation of cataracts and a lack of vitamin B2. Other symptoms of deficiency of riboflavin include cracked lips and tongue, increased sensitivity to light, and mouth lesions.

Those who may be deficient in this vitamin include people who habitually skip meals, refuse to eat liver or green vegetables, or follow a restrictive diet over a long period of time. Alcoholism may also lead to B2 deficiency. Vitamin B2 must be replaced daily.

Benefits

- aids in utilization of energy
- helps clear up lesions of the mouth, lips, skin, genitalia benefits vision, alleviates eye fatigue, prevents twilight blindness
- helps eliminate sore mouth, lips, tongue, skin, genitalia
- promotes healthy skin, nails, hair
- aids in growth and reproduction
- functions with other substances to metabolize carbohydrates, fats, proteins
- aids in stress situations
- helps eliminate dandruff
- assists in the uptake of iron and vitamin B6
- necessary for proper fetal development
- may help prevent cataracts
- may help control and treat carpal tunnel syndrome

Natural Sources

Liver, kidney, fish, eggs, cheese, milk, yeast, leafy green vegetables, brewer's yeast, blackstrap molasses, currants, avocados, nuts and beans

Deficiencies

Alopecia, blurred vision, cataracts, depression, dermatitis, dizziness, eyes (itching, burning, red), geographic tongue, growth retardation, pancreatic atrophy

VITAMIN B3 (Niacin)

Vitamin B3 is necessary for a healthy nervous system and proper brain function. A lack of this vitamin can cause negative personality changes. Niacin has been used to treat schizophrenia and other mental disorders such as anxiety, nervousness and depression. Several studies have also suggested that it may be beneficial in the treatment of epilepsy in conjunction with anti-convulsant drugs.

Vitamin B3 is also essential for the body to produce cortisone, thyroxine, insulin, and male and female sex hormones. Vitamin B3 is a vasodilator which can increase blood flow to the extremities. In addition, studies have shown that it is effective against certain type of carcinogens and may be useful in preventing some forms of cancer.

The body can usually produce its own vitamin B3, but only if it is receiving enough vitamins B1, B2, and B6. Alcoholics and severely malnourished individuals are prone to a vitamin B3 deficiency. B3 requirements are usually higher in individuals who have cancer, those taking oral contraceptives and anyone with a protein deficiency. The most obvious sign of a severe niacin deficiency is the disease Pellagra.

If you are taking extra vitamin B3, you may notice a flushing and itching of the skin—this is normal and should not last long. Vitamin B3 must be replaced daily.

Benefits

- combats pellagra, confusion, digestive difficulties, and blotched skin; relieves such symptoms as perceptual changes ("hearing things" or "seeing things" that aren't there)
- counteracts arteriosclerosis (hardening of the arteries)
- reduces cholesterol
- increases circulation and reduces high blood pressure
- helps prevent or make less severe migraine headaches
- promotes a healthy digestive system
- eliminates canker sores and improves skin's general appearance
- eases some attacks of diarrhea
- sometimes helps eliminate bad breath

Natural Sources

Liver, lean meat, kidney, fish, eggs, the white meat of poultry, whole wheat, yeast, wheat germ, roasted peanuts, avocados, dates, figs, prunes, potatoes, corn flour, broccoli, tomatoes, and carrots. (When using vegetable sources this vitamin can be lost in the cooking water. Steaming, baking or stir-frying vegetables is recommended.)

Deficiencies

Anorexia, nausea, canker sores, confusion, depression, dermatitis, diarrhea, crying jags, emotional, fatigue, halitosis (bad breath), headaches, indigestion, dyspepsia, insomnia, irritability, limb pains, memory loss, muscular weakness, skin eruptions/ eczema, diabetes, shock, allergic reactions, schizophrenia, arthritis

VITAMIN B5 (Pantothenic Acid)

Vitamin B5 is necessary in the production of various hormones. It is also used to build antibodies and to convert foods into useable energy. It helps in the production of new cells and the maintenance of normal growth and resistance to stress.

Pantothenic acid is also known as the anti-stress vitamin. It plays a key role in the formation of antibodies, the production of adrenal hormones, and the utilization of vitamins. Vitamin B5 also helps to convert fats, carbohydrates and proteins into useable energy. Pantothenic acid is required by body cells for normal growth and repair, and healthy functioning of the gastrointestinal tract relies on the presence of this vitamin. There is some evidence that vitamin B5 may also be useful in treating depression and anxiety disorders.

Some people who suffer from rheumatoid arthritis have significantly lower levels of pantothenic acid. In some cases, therapeutic doses of pantothenic acid have helped treat the stiffness and pain associated with arthritis.

In artificially induced deficiences, headache, fatigue, insomnia and nervouness occurred. These symptoms resulted from faulty adrenal gland function which helps the body cope with mental and physical stress. Pantothenic acid is needed for the adrenals.

Benefits

- strengthens adrenals
- helps control hypoglycemia
- aids in preventing duodenal ulcers
- fights infections and disease
- prevents fatigue
- aids in healing wounds
- speeds recovery after surgery
- reduces negative effects of antibiotics
- helps prevent blood and skin disorders
- eases pain of arthritis

Natural Sources

Meats, kidney, heart, liver, chicken, nuts, whole grains, wheat germ, bran, Brewer's yeast, broccoli, cauliflower, sweet potatoes, eggs, mushrooms, molasses, green vegetables, tomatoes, potatoes, beans, egg yolks, salt water fish

Deficiencies

Abdominal pain, alopecia, burning feet and hands, coordination impairment, depression, headaches, vertigo, leg muscle cramps, constipation, tendency toward hypoglycemia, arthritis, eczema, faintness, fatigue, hypotension, infections, insomnia, irritability, duodenal ulcers, impairment of hydrochloric acid secretion, stress, nausea and vomiting, nervousness, tachycardia, weakness, muscle spasms

VITAMIN B6 (Pyridoxine)

Vitamin B6 is primarily useful in assuring proper chemical balance in the blood and body tissues. It helps to maintain salt and water balances and is thus a natural diuretic. It is very useful in cases of edema (water retention) in the legs and certainly water retention around the heart. It certainly is necessary for the production of hydrochloric acid which is needed for digestion.

This vitamin is involved in the function of more body systems than any other vitamin, making it one of the most essential and utilized nutrients. It is involved in the maintenance of almost all bodily operations including: the metabolism of amino acids, absorption of fats and proteins, the production of red blood cells, RNA, and DNA, and is necessary in synthesizing hydrochloric acid. In addition, it activates enzymes, promotes antibody formation, and plays a significant role in cancer immunity and in the prevention of arteriosclerosis.

The nervous system depends on pyridoxine to prevent depression, irritability, dizziness and even brain abnormalities. Its presence in the body is essential for the production of serotonin, which plays a role in mood control. Recent studies have strongly suggested that vitamin B6 may prove very useful for women who suffer from PMS. In addition, it may also help to prevent oxalate kidney stones.

Those whose diets are high in protein and women who take birth control pills are likely to need extra vitamin B6. In addition, pregnant or nursing mothers require more pyridoxine and several studies indicate that some women may not be getting enough. There is always a B6 deficiency in carpal tunnel syndrome.

Benefits

- helps treat anemia
- alleviates nausea, specifically morning sickness
- controls cholesterol level in blood
- reduces muscle spasms, particularly cramps and numbness which occur at night
- promotes healthy skin, teeth, muscles, and nerves
- helps prevent kidney and gallstones
- builds resistance to ear infections
- eases air- and seasickness
- aids digestion
- helps lessen symptoms of PMS

- may be useful in treating carpal tunnel syndrome
- helps combat depression and other mental disorders

Natural Sources

Lean organ meats, liver, kidney, heart, milk, eggs, soybeans, nuts, yeast, wheat bran, wheat germ, cantaloupe, bananas, molasses, and leafy green vegetables, whole grains, cabbage, potatoes, peas, green peppers, salmon, cod

Deficiencies

Acne, alopecia, anemia, anorexia and nausea, arthritis, conjunctivitis, depression, dizziness, facial oiliness, fatigue, geographic tongue, mouth disorders, skin conditions, carpal tunnel syndrome, adrenal gland exhaustion, edema, hormonal imbalances, muscle pain, confusion, greenish tint to urine, joint swelling, menstrual and menopausal problems, kidney stones, impaired wound healing, irritability, nervousness, neurologic symptoms, seizures, stomatitis, stunted growth, weakness

VITAMIN B12 (Cyanocobalamin)

Vitamin B12 is actually a coenzyme that is necessary to metabolize fats and carbohydrates. Pernicious anemia is the most classic symptoms of a vitamin B12 deficiency. Vitamin B12 also assists in the proper digestion and absorption of foods. This vitamin also helps to prevent nerve damage, and promotes normal growth. Recent studies have suggested a possible link between dementia and low blood levels of vitamin B12. In addition, when this vitamin is combined with ascorbic acid, it has been shown to inhibit the formation of malignant cells in laboratory tests.

Vegetarians risk deficiency in vitamin B12 and so should supplement their diets with this vitamin. Women who are pregnant or nursing also benefit from additional B12. Anyone who suffers from any gastrointestinal disorder or uses nicotine may also suffer from a lack of vitamin B12. Elderly people sometime suffer from malabsorption which can also cause a lack of B12. Anti-gout medications, anticoagulant drugs and even potassium may block the assimilation of vitamin B12 in the digestive tract. Deficiency symptoms include: memory loss, hallucinations, eye disorders, anemia and digestive impairment.

Because it is sometimes difficult for the body to absorb B12, it should be combined with calcium. This vitamin is not stable if exposed to heat, acid or light, therefore, care is required during the cooking and storage of foods.

Vitamin B12 is effective in very small doses.

Benefits

- prevents anemia
- helps ease asthma
- promotes growth and increases appetite in children
- prevents eye damage, particularly from smoke or pollution
- increases energy
- relieves irritability
- maintains nervous system
- aids digestion
- helps improve concentration, memory, and balance
- a lack of this vitamin may be linked with dementia
- may be useful in combating depression and psychosis

Natural Sources

Liver, kidney, beef, saltwater fish, oysters, eggs, dairy products, lamb, clams, sardines, and tofu

Deficiencies

Achlorhydria, anemia, birth defects, constipation, brain damage, nervous disorders, lethargy, body odor, impairs function of small intestine, blood platelet function is impaired, allergies, insomnia, menstrual disturbances, apathy, weight loss, depression, dizziness, dyspnea (labored breathing), fatigue, GI upset, geographic tongue, headache, irritability, moodiness, numbness, palpitations, psychosis, spinal cord degeneration

VITAMIN B13 (Orotic Acid)

Very little research has yet been done on vitamin B13. Studies have found that orotic acid may be useful in the treatment of multiple sclerosis. In addition, it is believed that vitamin B13 may also facilitate the use of folic acid and vitamin B12. Properties of this vitamin make it beneficial for nervous system health and efficient functioning of the brain. A deficiency of this vitamin is thought to lead to liver disorders, cell degeneration and premature aging. Water and sunlight can deplete vitamin B13 stores. It is not currently available in the United States, but it can be obtained in Europe.

Benefits

- possible prevents some liver problems
- aids in treatment of multiple sclerosis
- helps prevent premature aging
- helps promote efficient brain and nervous system function
- retards cell degeneration

Natural Sources

Root vegetables (carrots, potatoes, turnips, etc.), whey, liquid from curdled milk, yogurt, and some fruits

VITAMIN B15 (Pangamic Acid)

The essential requirement for vitamin B15 has not been proved. It is enthusiastically used in Russia, but the U.S. Food and Drug

Administration has given some resistance to its sale in the United States. Pangamic acid helps to improve the body's ability to use oxygen by improving blood circulation. It also plays a role in the metabolism of protein, fat and carbohydrates. Vitamin B15 also stimulates both the glandular and nervous systems and is believed to help prevent premature aging. It also helps in stabilizing nervous disorders. In addition, it keeps fat particles from accumulating in the blood, promotes tissue healing, helps to protect against carbon monoxide poisoning and other carcinogenic pollutants. Some studies have shown that Vitamin B15 acts as a preventative substance against cancer. Using alcohol, coffee and laxatives can deplete vitamin B15 stores.

Some people become slightly nauseated for a little while after starting to take B15, but this usually lasts only a few days. Taking the vitamin after the day's largest meal helps ease this nausea.

B15 acts more effectively if taken together with vitamins A and E. Russians recommend taking 50 mg. three times a day for 90 days, cutting back then to one a day.

Benefits

- stops the craving for alcohol
- speeds recovery from fatigue
- extends cell life span
- protects against pollutants
- helps lower cholesterol level
- aids in protein synthesis
- increases immunity to infections
- relieves symptoms of angina and asthma
- helps prevent cirrhosis
- aids in easing hangovers
- helps control high blood pressure
- aids in treating hepatitis and cirrhosis of the liver
- eases headaches
- mental disorders

Natural Sources

Whole grains, whole brown rice, pumpkin seeds, sesame seeds, Brewer's yeast, liver, sunflower seeds, and apricot kernels

Deficiencies

Premature aging, diminished cell oxygenation, asthma, neuritis, emphysema, liver diseases, fatigue, glaucoma, angina, hypertension, autism, schizophrenia, heart disease, glandular and nervous disorders

VITAMIN B17 (Laetrile)

Vitamin B17 is very controversial. It has been rejected by the U.S. Food and Drug Administration, and its use in cancer treatment is legal only in part of the United States. It contains natural cyanide (benzaldehyde) which is believed to kill cancer cells. It is because of this cyanide content that laetrile has been banned by the FDA. Regardless of its current standing, there is a significant number of health care providers that still advocate that laetrile does indeed help to prevent and control cancer. They believe that laetrile literally poisons malignant cells without damaging healthy tissue. Laetrile was also found to increase appetite and decrease pain in cancer patients, therefore improving their overall outlook and enabling them to gain weight. Laetrile also stimulates the production of hemoglobin, thus boosting red blood cell count. It has been produced commercially in Germany.

Massive doses of B17 should never be taken all at once. It is better to take small doses at different times during the day. It is recommended to take in addition to B17 large doses of vitamin A (in emulsion form) and large doses of enzymes. Excessive amounts of this vitamin can be dangerous. The use of alcohol and coffee deplete vitamin B17 stores.

Benefits

- may aid in preventing or controlling some cancers
- may help to control sickle-cell anemia

Natural Sources

The pits of apricots, cherries, peaches, plums, nectarines, apples, almonds, peas, broad beans, papayas, alfalfa seeds, alfalfa leaves, berries, sorghum, millet, buckwheat and various types of seeds

Deficiencies

A lack of this nutrient is thought by many scientists to cause cancer.

VITAMIN B FACTORS (Inositol)

Inositol is a nutrient which we are able to synthesize in our bodies. As a result, inositol is not considered an essential vitamin, nevertheless its value should not be minimized. Inositol is involved in the body's use of fats and cholesterol and is needed for the proper transportation and metabolism of fats. In laboratory studies, inositol has been shown to prevent or lessen the build up of abnormal amounts of fats in the liver. Inositol may also have been required to produce phospholipids which are necessary for the digestion and absorption of fats and the efficient uptake of fatty acids by the cells. Inositol is also believed to reduce blood levels of cholesterol by assisting in the production of lecithin. It also helps to stimulate the normal growth of cells in the bone marrow and eye membranes.

Inositol seems to be most effective when taken together with other vitamins, particularly vitamin E, choline, and biotin.

Inositol appears to be important in the proper function of the heart, eyes, and brain. Ingesting large amounts of caffeine, alcohol, water and taking sulfa drugs deplete inositol stores in the body. In addition, prolonged exposure to certain insect poisons may cause a shortage of this nutrient.

Benefits

- prevents eczema
- promotes healthy hair and helps prevent hair loss

- regulates cholesterol levels and aids in treatment of arthersclerosis
- aids in redistribution of body fat
- builds resistance to cirrhosis of the liver
- helps in treatment of nerve damage from some types of muscular dystrophy
- counteracts negative effects of caffeine
- constipation
- helps to prevent glaucoma
- combats gall bladder disease
- works to prevent and treat obesity
- produces a gradual lowering of blood pressure in mild hypertension
- is a sedative—is used in problems of sleep including insomnia
- is known as nature's anxiety fighter

Natural Sources

Organ meats (liver, heart, brains), peanuts, dried lima beans, yeast, molasses, corn, nuts, wheat germ, raisins, cantaloupe, grapefruit, cabbage, oranges, soybeans, sesame seeds, whole wheat bread, oatmeal, brewer's yeast and lecithin

Deficiencies

Alopecia, poor appetite, constipation, eczema, hypercholesterolemia, cardiovascular disease, insomnia, nephritis, anxiety, stress, fatty liver, dermatitis.

VITAMIN B FACTORS (Choline)

Choline is used by the body to produce acetylcholine, which is a neurotransmitter found in the brain. It is vital that an adequate supply of choline is found in the body in order to maintain healthy nerve function. Choline is also necessary for proper gallbladder regulation, liver function and lecithin formation. Like inositol, it also helps to reduce the accumulation of excess fats in the liver and participates in fat and cholesterol regulation.

Choline has also been found to strengthen weak capillaries and can help to prevent the formation of gallstones. It is vital to the proper digestion of fatty foods and is needed for the storage of minerals, especially calcium and vitamin A.

Choline is necessary in liver development and in maintaining the functions of both liver and kidney.

It is also required in the thin covering of nerve fibers—a deficiency of choline and can damage the nerves and so impair body functions. It has been shown that a deficit of choline may play a role in the development of certain neurologic disorders such as Huntington's chorea, Parkinson's disease and Alzheimer's disease. Lecithin, a natural source of choline, has been used to successfully treat cases of tardive dyskinesia a condition characterized by uncontrolled facial twitches.

Taking estrogen, sulfa drugs, alcohol, and excessive sugar and water deplete choline in the body.

Benefits

- helps control cholesterol
- sustains healthy nerves, kidneys, liver
- maintains muscles
- helps control blood pressure
- aids those nerve impulses that effect memory
- assists liver in eliminating poisons from the blood
- helps to treat hepatitis
- may be useful in preventing or decreasing attacks of multiple sclerosis
- plays a role in preventing arteriosclerosis and heart trouble
- may help to prevent Alzheimer's disease, Huntington's chorea and Parkinson's disease

Natural Sources

Organ meats, egg yolks, yeast, wheat germ, peanuts or peanut butter, green leafy vegetables, rice bran, various seeds, soybeans, liver, peas, brewer's yeast, lecithin, and turnip greens, and fish

Deficiencies

Cirrhosis of the liver, hemorrhages of the kidneys, high blood pressure, atherosclerosis, eczema, hypertension, muscular weakness, loss of memory, bleeding stomach ulcers, heart palpitations, dizziness, headaches, cardiac symptoms, growth retardation, myasthenia gravis and other neurological diseases

VITAMIN B FACTORS (Folic Acid)

Folic acid works with vitamin B12 in the body and is crucial for the proper metabolism of amino acids and the production of proteins. It is vital for the normal synthesis of RNA and DNA which determines the healthy division of cells and regeneration of body tissues. For this reason, the requirement of folic acid is dramatically increased during illness, injury or after surgery.

Folic acid is also considered a brain food and is needed to produce and maintain certain brain chemicals that can determine mood changes and mental health. In some cases, folic acid has been effective in the treatment of uterine cervical conditions that are considered precancerous.

In addition, folic acid helps to regulate fetal development of nerve cells and is vital for the normal growth and development of the fetus.

Folic acid is most effective when taken with vitamin B12. In turn, it is necessary for the full effectiveness of vitamins A, D, E, and K.

Those who should increase their folic acid intake include people who take large doses of vitamin C, women who are pregnant (particularly just before delivery) or nursing, women who take birth control pills, and person who drink alcoholic beverages. Other drugs that have been shown to increase the body's requirement of folic acid are: aspirin, nitrous oxide, anticonvulsants, diuretics and sulfasalazine used to treat bowel disorders. Classic symptoms that a deficiency of folic acid exists include: mutated red blood cell anemia, irritability, insomnia, weakness and pallor. Sixty-eight percent of folic acid is lost when wheat is processed into white flour.

Benefits

- helps prevent anemia
- improves lactation
- aids in reducing pain
- protects against intestinal parasites and food poisoning
- sometimes helps delay the graying of hair (when used with pantothenic acid and PABA)
- increases appetite in those who are run down
- promotes healthy-looking skin
- helps prevent canker sores
- aids in atherosclerosis
- may help treat depression and other mental disorders
- may delay the growth of precancerous cell in the female cervix
- helps prevent birth defects such as spina bifida

Natural Sources

Liver, egg yolks, yeast, bran, avocados, pumpkins, cantaloupe, apricots, brewer's yeast, whole wheat, dark rye flour, deep green leafy vegetables, carrots, fresh mushrooms, sprouts, yogurt, and soybeans

Deficiencies

Anemia, anorexia, apathy, birth defects, (spina bifida, hydroencephalocoele), GI upsets/diarrhea, dyspepsia, chronic fatigue, geographic tongue, atherosclerosis, gout, slow development or poor learning ability, psoriasis, growth retardation, headache, insomnia, memory loss, paranoia, vitiligo, weakness, headaches

VITAMIN C (Ascorbic Acid)

Vitamin C plays a significant role in several key functions of the body. Its importance to the proper functioning of the immune system cannot be overestimated. Over the last few years, studies have confirmed that vitamin C helps to increase resistance to infectious diseases including cancer. Increased dosages of vitamin C have been found to stimulate the production of white blood cells which fight off bacterial and viral invaders in the body.

Vitamin C is also considered an antioxidant that is vital to tissue growth and repair, adrenal gland function and the maintenance of healthy gums. Another important role of vitamin C concerns its ability to help cope with all kinds of physical and mental stressors. In addition, this vitamin plays a primary role in the formation of collagen which is essential to healthy bones and teeth.

Vitamin C is essential for the body to produce collagen, which is the substance that bonds cells together. Maintaining vitamin C in your body therefore helps preserve and mend the connective tissues (tendons and cartilage - including the cartilage between spinal discs), bones, muscles, and blood vessels. Vitamin C also helps to protect against the harmful effects of pollution, bruising and blood clotting. It promotes tissue healing and assists in interferon production. Its presence is required for the metabolism of folic acid, tyrosine and phenylalanine.

There is growing evidence that vitamin C and vitamin E work together more effectively when combined in extending antioxidant activity. While vitamin C is not considered a cure for colds, taking it at the onset of symptoms can make the cold substantially milder. Vitamin C can also act to help prevent high blood pressure and hardening of the arteries which can lead to heart attack or stroke.

Vitamin C also helps the body use iron. Dr. Linus Pauling, two time Nobel prize winner, has documented curing cancer in fifty seven cases considered to be incurable. He used vitamin C in the amounts of 10 to 30,000 milligrams a day in these individuals to achieve success.

You need extra vitamin C if you:
- smoke.
- take aspirin often.
- live or work in a city or other environment with carbon. monoxide in the air.
- take birth control pills.

Vitamin C must be replaced daily. The body cannot manufacture vitamin C, therefore it must be obtained through certain foods or supplements. Most vitamin C is lost in the urine. Ester C is a new form of the vitamin that enters the tissues at a much faster rate and may be more useful for persons suffering from chronic infections such as cancer and AIDS. Vitamin C is unquestionably a marvelous nutrient and unfortunately, most of us are at a high risk of not getting the amounts we need. The addition of bioflavonoids to vitamin C is believed by many to enhance the potency of the vitamin in all regards. Natural sources of vitamin C are preferable.

Benefits

- prevents scurvy
- helps prevent or make less severe the common cold
- promotes healing of wounds, burns, and bone fractures
- increases resistance to infections, fatigue, and low temperatures
- aids in prevention of internal bleeding
- helps guard against anemia
- maintains solid bones and teeth
- promotes healthy gums
- helps relieve back problems and related discomforts
- acts as a mild diuretic
- helps body meet various stresses
- encourages healing after surgery
- aids in decreasing cholesterol level in the blood
- reduces discomforts of allergies
- gives a high resistance to cancer
- fights also against cataracts, cystitis, pyorrhea, aging, diabetes, and gallstones

Natural Sources

Citrus fruits (oranges, grapefruit, lemons, limes, tomatoes), fresh fruits and vegetables, green leafy vegetables, broccoli, cauliflower, berries, cantaloupe, potatoes, acerola cherry juice, black currants, horseradish, raw red and green peppers, and rose hips.

Deficiencies

Bleeding gums/loose teeth, depression, tiredness, easy bruising, irritability, joint pain, impaired wound healing.

VITAMIN D

Vitamin D in some respects is not considered to be a true vitamin in that in its active form it is considered a hormone and our bodies can synthesize it from sunlight.

Vitamin D is necessary for the body to build calcium in the bones. It is also required to release the calcium for the body's use. Because of this, vitamin D deficiency is usually related to calcium deficiency conditions. Vitamin D plays a vital role in helping to prevent osteoporosis, rickets, hypocalcemia and immune system deficiencies. When the body is low on vitamin D, the bones can become brittle or deformed, the teeth underdeveloped and overall growth can be stunted in children. Calcium and magnesium should always be given along with vitamin D to help the body maintain bone mass which is often lost in post menopausal women.

Recent studies have shown that vitamin D, when taken with calcium, may offer some anticancer properties. In addition, a lack of this vitamin can predispose some people to high blood pressure. In some instances, therapeutic doses of vitamin D have proven beneficial in treating psoriasis and mood disorders. It also may improve muscle strength and stamina.

We can receive vitamin D directly from the sunshine as well as through diet. Those whose clothing, environment, or work schedules limit their exposure to the sun should probably increase the vitamin D in their diets. It should be noted that once a suntan is established, the skin no longer absorbs vitamin D from the sun. Ingesting mineral oil, exposure to smog, the use of barbiturates, steroids, sleeping pills and some anticonvulsants can deplete vitamin D in the body.

Women who are pregnant or nursing need extra vitamin D, as do children who are still growing.

Benefits

- prevents rickets
- helps prevent osteomalacia and some irregularities in heartbeat
- builds strong bones and teeth
- aids in producing blood plasma
- is effective in treatment of keratoconus
- relieves chronic conjunctivitis
- prevents colds when taken with vitamins A and C
- helps body use calcium, phosphorus and vitamin A
- may help treat psoriasis
- helps to build up muscle strength
- is useful in the treatment of acne

Natural Sources

Dairy products, ultraviolet sun rays, egg yolk, fish liver oils, sardines, herring, salmon, tuna, and spinach

Deficiencies

Burning in the mouth and throat, osteomalacia, rickets, nervousness, myopia, insomnia, diarrhea, fragile and broken bones, osteoporosis, constipation, cramps, fatigue, arthritis, kidney diseases, poor bone and tooth formation

VITAMIN E

Vitamin E, like vitamin C is also considered an antioxidant. In this regard it is thought to help prevent cancer and heart disease. Recent studies suggest that vitamin E may play a vital role in the biological functions that relate to the aging process. There is some evidence that this vitamin may slow down aging by prolonging the life span of cells in the body.

Vitamin E also improves circulation, tissue regeneration and is useful in treating fibrocystic disease of the breasts and PMS. This vitamin also promotes healing and reduces scarring, assists in reducing blood pressure and may help to prevent cataracts.

The presence of vitamin E may also help to protect the body from a variety of carcinogens and toxins including, mercury, lead, benzene, nitrites, cigarette smoke and polluted air. In addition, there is evidence to support that taking vitamin E can help minimize the toxic effect of anyone undergoing cancer chemotherapy.

There is also data that indicates that vitamin E has the capability of increasing HDL cholesterol levels which is a form of cholesterol that actually protects the body against heart disease.

Vitamin E acts to control the unsaturated fatty acids in the body; it affects virtually all body tissues. Vitamin E is more potent when taken together with selenium. Vitamin E boosts the action of vitamin A.

Those who drink chlorinated water and women who are pregnant, nursing, taking birth control pills, or going through the menopause need extra vitamin E.

In Europe, tests were done with human beings and animals and it was found that if vitamin E is taken away from the human being completely, reproduction would stop. This vitamin E is considered a necessity for having good healthy children. There are also studies done in Canada showing that 400 IU of vitamin E taken daily lowered cardiac risks by more than 50 percent. Athletes have taken vitamin E for years to increase their endurance.

Vitamin E may be applied directly in treatment of wounds or other skin disorders.

Vitamin E should be replaced regularly. The body needs zinc in order to ensure proper levels of vitamin E in the bloodstream. Vitamin E deficiency symptoms include anemia, neurological disturbances, and capillaries that break easily.

Benefits

- strengthens and protects reproductive, muscular, circulatory, skeletal, and nervous systems
- improves circulation
- helps prevent arteriosclerosis and blood clots

- useful in treating gangrene, nephritis, rheumatic fever, purpura, retinitis, diabetes mellitus, congenital heart disease, phlebitis
- prevents or lessens scar tissue, both internal and external, and so is helpful after surgery or heart attack
- aids healing of wounds, burns, chronic ulcers, and some skin diseases
- protects respiratory system from pollution
- increases fertility
- prevents premature aging
- improves endurance
- acts as mild diuretic (and may therefore lower blood pressure)
- helps prevent miscarriage
- counteracts fatigue
- strengthens heart
- carries oxygen
- goes straight to placenta

Natural Sources

Wheat germ, vegetable oils, peanuts, whole-grain cereals, green leafy vegetables, broccoli, spinach, eggs, peas, corn, dessicated liver, organ meats, brown rice and sweet potatoes

Deficiencies

RBC fragility, gait disturbances, infertility, dermatitis, alopecia, malabsorption, muscular dystrophy, atherosclerosis, thrombosis, ruptured blood vessels, anemia, angina pectoris, hemorrhoids, varicose veins, fat deposits in the muscle, shrinkage of connective tissue

VITAMIN F (Unsaturated Essential Fatty Acids)

Fatty degeneration diseases today kill over 75 percent of the people living in the affluent, industrialized nations before they reach 70 years of age. To get at the root of the problem, we must investigate the supply of fatty foods and their sources, availability and benefits as utilizable health sustaining providers of proper nutrient. We need to best sustain them in regard to fatty foods and their enhancement of good health so as to avoid fatty degenerative diseases.

We find that there are two Essential fatty acids. Essential meaning that these fatty acids are essential to life and are not manufactured by the body from any substance or substances and must be provided to our bodies in our foods. The names of these two fatty acids are linoleic acid and linolenic acid. Another name is vitamin F.

EFAs function is to strengthen cell membranes and promote the growth of muscles and bones. Therapeutically, they are used to thin the blood, inhibit clotting and improve cholesterol profiles. These essential fatty acids can aid in the prevention of heart disease if provided in sufficient quantities and quality. EFAs are anti-inflammatory and useful in the treatment of arthritis, allergies and asthma. Essential fatty acids are also known as unsaturated fatty acids.

Unsaturated fatty acids are vital in lowering blood pressure, controlling cholesterol levels and in reducing the risk of heart disease and stroke. Essential fatty acids are vital for maintaining normal function of the adrenal and thyroid glands, for proper blood coagulation and for healthy hair and skin cells.

Vitamin F stimulates the conversion of carotene into vitamin A and provides protection against the harmful effects of X-rays. Essential fatty acids play a vital part in the necessary utilization of fats by the body. The unsaturated fatty acids, by providing the body with fats in a form which can be used, aids in burning up the saturated fats. Of the two essential fatty acids, Linolenic and Linoleic acid, Linoleic is the most essential.

Flaxseed oil contains both essential fatty acids in large quantities and has an abundance of the more rare linolenic acid. It also has anti-estrogen activity derived from its fiber, called lignins. Urine of vegetarian women have an above normal supply of lignins and thus have a reduced risk of developing breast cancer. The contents of stabilized flaxseed is higher in lignin's than in any other food with buckwheat and wheat following and vegetables containing the smallest amount. Dr. Budwig, the world¿s leading expert on the therapeutic uses of flax oil, uses it with good success for enemas in cases of colon cancer and bowel obstructions. Flaxseed oil has the highest content, twice as much Omega-3 as fish oil. Linseed oil as used in paint is made from flaxseed but as processed and stored is rancid and poison to humans. It is estimated that over 80 percent of the United State's population probably has an Omega-3 deficiency. Omega-3 is known to naturally thin the blood thus making unnecessary the use of aspirin as a blood thinner in potential heart problems and will aid in cleaning out the heart and other blood vessels that clogged arteries commonly found in those who partake of the usual bill of fair on our tables from food provided in our food markets. Blood clots can cause heart attacks and strokes, but carefully extracted and stored flaxseed oil prevents blood clotting by reducing blood platelets from clumping.

The three essential fatty acids are 1) Alpha linolenic Acid (Omega 3), 2) Linoleic Acid (Omega 6) and 3) Oleic Acid (Omega 9). Some of the functions performed by these essential fatty acids include:

1. Metabolism of cholesterol and triglycerides
2. Cell membrane formation
3. Energy production
4. Normal brain development and function
   (specific to Omega 3)
5. Involved in the function of the immune system

In 1899, Rosenfeld demonstrated that the consumption of animal fats (high in saturated and low in the essential fatty acids) causes obesity and fatty degeneration of the inner organs. In 1902, Rosenfeld showed that a high carbohydrate, low protein diet results in fat deposition as does a high carbohydrate, high protein diet. However, when essential fatty acids containing fats are added, less fat deposition occurs with better food utilization and energy production taking place. Fats high in essential fatty acids help one stay slim.

Essential fatty acids increase the metabolic rate, helping to mobilize and burn excess saturated fats. This is vital to improved health and the prevention of conditions caused by obstructed blood passages.

With the sufficient intake of essential fatty acids, one of its role in loosing excess fat is in the loss of the craving for more food which results when the body's need for essential fatty acids is satisfied. The hunger mechanism is set up to shut off only when the nutrient needs of the body are fulfilled. A diet lacking in essential substances leads to continuing hunger, overeating and weight gain.

RECOMMENDATIONS ON THE USE OF DIETARY FATS

1. LOWER TOTAL FAT CONSUMPTION
   (Obvious sources: margarine, shortening, butter, refined vegetable oils, hidden fats (hamburgers, cheese—except low-fat cheeses, salad dressings, potato chips, fried foods)
2. INCREASE ESSENTIAL FATTY ACID CONSUMPTION
3. LOWER REFINED SUGARS AND STARCHES
   (catsup, ice cream, canned vegetables which are sweetened, macaroni, pastas, enriched flours, noodles)
4. LOWER HARD FATS AND CHOLESTEROL
   (Example: One month on a strictly vegetarian diet (no meat, no eggs, no dairy) can bring down the blood cholesterol level from 260 mg. to 160 mg. The average blood cholesterol level of a heart attack patient is 244 mg.).
5. INCREASE FIBER, VITAMINS AND MINERALS
   (Fiber such as apples, potatoes, beets, carrots, okra, bananas and oats carry bile acids and cholesterol out of the body. Several vitamins and minerals are required to protect the essential fatty acids from destruction by oxygen and free radicals. Vitamins A/beta carotene, C and E with selenium and the minerals zinc, B-complex, chromium, a high potency vitamin/mineral supplement, but add extra vitamin C and E).
6. AVOID ALTERED FATS
   (Avoid hydrogenated oil products like shortenings, margarines, bakery products, candies, fries, deep-fried foods and processed convenience foods. Use raw seeds and nuts which are the prime choice for health-giving fats and oils).
7. MINIMIZE DRUGS AND AVOID FOOD ADDITIVES
   (Avoid the man-made, highly processed, artifically colored and flavored foods and return to fresh fruits and vegetables, whole grains and seeds and the wild meats (especially fish).

8. EXERCISE
(We need exercise. The body is made for activity. Lack of exercise results in stagnation and poor metabolism of fats, carbohydrates and proteins. If our only exercise is the grinding movement of the jaws, the movement of our hands from plate to mouth, and the push away from the table, that's not enough. Regular activity is extremely important for the maintenance of health).

Erasmus, Udo. *Fats and Oils.* Alive Books, British Columbia, 1986, Pgs. 317-322.

As a caution, it should be known that both linoleic and linolenic acid are sensitive to destruction by light, oxygen and high temperatures and their absence in the system is fatal. Severe problems are caused by the deficiency of essential oils in every cell, tissue and organ and is related to degenerative diseases.

It must be remembered to take vitamin E with vitamin F for best absorption in the system. Linoleic acid utilization requires niacin, B-6, vitamin C, zinc and magnesium to work efficiently.

Essential fatty acids absorb sunlight through the skin. The absorption of light energy increases their ability to react with oxygen by about 1,000 fold, and makes them chemically very active. Essential fatty acids attract oxygen.

Essential fatty acids due to their negative charges, are responsible for a number of activities vital to life. Molecules repel each other due to this charge, they spread out in a very thin layer over surfaces, and do not form aggregations (a clustering or coming together of substances, i.e., clumping together of blood cells, especially platelets or red cells). Surface activity provides the power in the biological system, to carry toxins substances to the surface of the skin, intestinal tract, kidneys, or lungs where these substances are discarded.

- Essential fatty acids help in maintaining a uniform healthy body temperature.
- Essential fatty acids are necessary for maintaining the insulation of nerves, the use of fat in cushioning and protecting tissues and the creation of stored energy.

- Essential fatty acids are precursors of prostaglandin's, which must be present for dilating blood vessels and in the healthy regulation of arterial pressure, metabolizing cholesterol, activating T-lymphocyte, protecting against platelet aggregation, controlling abnormal cell proliferation, and other functions.

Benefits

- prevents eczema and acne
- aids in weight reduction
- helps control cholesterol levels
- encourages healthy hair and skin
- provides some protection against negative effects of x-rays
- helps to control psoriasis
- aids in the prevention of arthritis
- may reduce the growth rate of breast cancer
- encourages normal blood clotting
- helps ensure proper brain function

Oil of Evening Primrose contains 72 percent linoleic acid. Linoleic acid is the major essential fatty acid with Oil of Evening Primrose containing only small amounts of the non-essential fatty acids. Oil of Evening Primrose contains 9 percent gamma linolenic acid, present in only a limited number of other plant seeds. The other main source of GLA is human mother,s milk present in sufficient amounts when the mother has sufficient intake of foods containg GLA. GLA is the first product in the chain of biochemical functions for the vital transformation of the main essential fatty acid, linoleic acid into prostaglandins.

- Black currant oil is higher in the level of GLA than that found in Evening Primrose Oil.
- Black currant oil is a rich source of vitamin C, B and rutin.
- Black currant seed oil provides essential fatty acids and is high in prostaglandins. It is the highest source of gamma-linolenic acid. It stimulates the immune response and has anti-viral and anti-inflammatory properties.

- Zinc is absolutely necessary, for the conversion of linoleic acid to gamma-linoleic acid.
- Zinc, vitamin C, vitamins B3 (niacin) and pyroxidine (B6) are co-factors in the body‚s conversion of GLA to prostaglandin.
- A functional deficiency of essential fatty acids has been postulated to cause abnormal sensitivity to prolactin and premenstrual syndrome (PMS).

FISH OILS (Omega-3 EPA)

There are some fish oils which, when taken on a regular basis, promotes clean arteries and the absence of fatty degeneration diseases. EPA (eicosapentaenoic acid) is a normal constituent of special human tissues, such as brain cells, synapses (nerve relay stations), retina, inner ear, adrenals and sex glands—the active tissues of the body.

EPA can be manufactured by the healthy human body, albeit slowly, from the essential fatty acid, linolenic acid, which is found in flax seeds, pumpkin seeds, soybeans and walnuts. However, many degenerative conditions impair the body's ability to make EPA. Fish oils, being highly unsaturated, will not aggregate, so it will help disperse aggregations of the saturated fatty acids, which like to stick together. Thus EPA keeps deposits of saturated fatty acids and cholesterol from glueing up our arteries and platelets from becoming sticky which can then lower blood pressure by 10 points.

EPA is also important because it is the fatty acid out of which the body produces prostaglandins.

LECITHIN

Lecithin is vital to the function of every living cell in the body. The composition of cell membranes is largely made up of lecithin. Lecithin is crucial to protect cells from the damage which results from oxidation. Lecithin helps to regulate the metabolism of fat and cholesterol and significantly prevents it from sticking to artery walls. It functions to disperse and remove fats from the body. For this reason, it is vital that elderly people get adequate supplies of this nutrient to prevent arteriosclerosis. In addition, lecithin helps to fight infections by increasing cell resistance to infection. It also increases brain function, promotes energy and can help to repair liver damage caused by alcoholism.

Lecithin also offers some promise for victims of chronic viral disorders such as herpes or AIDS and immune disorders associated with aging. Lecithin also facilitates the absorption of thiamine by the liver and vitamin A in the intestines. Taking lecithin before eating can help to absorb fat-soluble vitamins and to more efficiently digest fats. Unquestionably, all vital organs and arteries benefit from the inclusion of lecithin in the diet. All the nerve endings in the body, including the spinal column are bathed in a solution of lecithin. For instance, the patient who dies of multiple sclerosis, they find that the myelin sheath is destroyed and the nerve endings are frayed, but they find no lecithin in all the nerve endings that are supposed to be bathed in a solution of lecithin. There are some men who have what they call a dry ejaculation which is very painful. The sperm is carried in a solution of lecithin and if lecithin is taken, generally this problem of dry ejaculation is taken care of. Sciatic nerve problems can be relieved generally by taking up to 25 lecithin capsules a day. Recurring of hemorrhoidal problems is caused by a deficiency of lecithin. Women who take lecithin during pregnancy have their cells hold their elasticity, thus returning to their original shape much easier after delivery.

Lecithin becomes rancid very easily and should be kep refrigerated at all times. If it becomes rancid, it can do more harm than good. One of the safest ways of taking lecithin is in the form of gelatin capsules as they have been hermetically sealed, giving extra protection against the problem of rancidity.

Benefits

- breaks down fat and cholesterol
- brain food
- lowers blood pressure

- increases gamma globulin in the blood
- helps fight infection
- skin disturbances such as eczema, acne and psoriasis
- softens aging skin
- natural tranquilizer
- sexual aid
- helpful in weight loss
- helpful in assimilation of vitamins A and E
- combination of vitamin E and Lecithin found useful in lowering the requirements of insulin in diabetics

Natural Sources

Major sources of Lecithin are soybeans, though traces are also found in all vegetable oils, such as corn and wheat germ oil. Soybean is most desirable because of its high protein content and availability.

Deficiencies

Nerve degeneration, cholesterol problems, chronic viral disorders, herpes, AIDS, immune disorders, aging, atherosclerosis

VITAMIN H (Biotin)

Biotin is an important coenzyme that is technically not a true vitamin because it is produced in the body by intestinal bacteria. Biotin contributes to cell growth, fatty acid synthesis, and in the proper utilization of fats, carbohydrates and proteins. It also helps to ensure that B-complex vitamins are assimilated properly.

Adequate quantities of biotin or vitamin H are necessary for healthy hair and skin. In some men, biotin is believed to prevent or slow baldness. Vitamin H also promotes healthy nerve tissue, bone marrow and sweat glands and all other secreting glands. This nutrient is also involved in male sex hormone production, and in fatty acid functions.

Vitamin H helps the liver produce lipids (fats) and promotes the conversion of food into energy. Vitamin H is necessary to utilize vitamin C. Raw egg whites counteract vitamin H, so those who eat or drink mixtures containing raw egg should increase their vitamin H. True deficiencies of biotin are rare because it is produced in the body, however if a malfunction occurs, symptoms include: dermatitis, hair loss, nausea, decreased appetite, high blood cholesterol and depression. Symptoms of a biotin deficiency mimic those of Alzheimer's disease in some cases. Some people who require dialysis may need extra supplements of biotin or vitamin H. Consuming rancid fats or saccharin may inhibit the absorption of biotin. The use of sulfa drugs or other antibiotics may interfere in the availability of biotin to body cells. There is no RDA for biotin at this time.

Benefits

- helps prevent eczema
- eases muscle pain
- aids metabolism
- helps prevent baldness and graying of hair
- builds resistance to some allergies
- alleviates or prevents exhaustion
- contributes to proper production of male sex hormone
- promotes efficient assimilation of B-complex vitamins
- contributes to health of all secreting glands

Natural Sources

Green leafy vegetables, nuts, fruits, unrefined rice, egg yolks, liver, kidney, milk, brewer's yeast, wheat germ, sprouts, molasses, yogurt, chicken, lamb, pork, salt water fish and rice bran

Deficiencies

Gray skin color, sore tongue, depression, anorexia, insomnia, anemia, muscle pain, impairment of fat metabolism, nausea, lethargy, baldness and gray hair, exzema, dry skin, fatigue, nervous system disturbances, dermatitis

VITAMIN K

Vitamin K is found in foods but because it is also produced by bacteria in the intestines, it is not considered a vitamin in the strict sense of the word. The most important function of vitamin K is the role it plays in the synthesis of blood clotting factors (prothrombin) in the body. Interestingly, the way that many rodent poisons work is by counteracting the effects of vitamin K, causing uncontrolled bleeding.

Several recent studies have also linked this vitamin with the prevention of osteoporosis. People who have unusually low levels of vitamin K may be susceptible to developing osteoporosis. Vitamin K is also influential in affecting behavior, and helps to protect the liver from toxins such as lead. It is required to some degree to convert carbohydrates into glucose.

Deficiencies of vitamin K are rare since it is found in a number of foods and is readily made in the body. If a bowel obstruction or malabsorption exists, stores of the vitamin can become depleted. Frequently, vitamin K is administered to people with blood clotting disorders prior to surgery. When combined with vitamin C it can be effective in helping to prevent hemorrhage. Taking antibiotics interferes with the absorption of vitamin K.

Besides its uses in the human body, vitamin K works as an excellent preservative for food. It does not alter the taste or appearance of the food it preserves.

Benefits

- helps prevent colitis
- promotes adequate blood clotting
- reduces susceptibility to nose bleeds
- works to counteract nausea in pregnant women
- reduces excessive menstrual flow
- prevents internal hemorrhaging
- aids in treating snakebite
- helps relieve pain
- may help to prevent osteoporosis

- works to minimize bruising
- may play a role in controlling erratic behavior

Natural Sources

Yogurt, green leafy vegetables, root vegetables (carrots, potatoes, turnips), alfalfa, safflower oil, soybean oil, kelp, egg yolks, liver, legumes, blackstrap molasses, and sprouts

Deficiencies

Delayed blood clotting, internal bleeding, subcutaneous hemorrhages, osteoporosis

VITAMIN P (Bioflavonoids)

Technically bioflavonoids are not vitamins although they are sometimes referred to as vitamin P. They are now accepted as antioxidants and are naturally found in the white portion of the peeling of citrus fruits. Bioflavonoids enhance the absorption of vitamin C and should be taken together. In addition, bioflavonoids strengthen capillary walls which can prevent varicose veins, bruising and hemorrhages. Bioflavonoids are routinely used for athletic injuries to prevent bruising and the formation of bumps.

Bioflavonoids have been found to also have antibiotic-like levels. Because they have a powerful anti-inflammatory capability, they may be useful in the treatment of arthritis. Some studies have suggested that when taken with vitamin C, bioflavonoids reduce the symptoms of oral herpes. In both humans and animals, bioflavonoids were shown to counteract cataract formation.

Bromelain and quercetin are bioflavonoids that have been used in the treatment of asthma and allergies. The body cannot produce bioflavonoids and it must be supplied in dietary forms. Smoking, ingesting aspirin, alcohol, cortisone, and antibiotics can deplete bioflavonoid supplies in the body.

Vitamin P is essential for the proper absorption and use of vitamin C. These two vitamins work together to strengthen capillaries and connective tissues. When you buy *natural* vitamin C; you usually get vitamin P as well.

Two well-known members of this Bioflavonoid complex are Rutin and Hesperidin. One of the richest sources of bioflavonoids is known as Pycnogenol.

Benefits

- prevents bruising
- helps treat edema and dizziness which result from inner ear infections
- builds resistance to infections
- prevents bleeding gums
- helps prevent miscarriage
- helps to build immunity to cancer
- eases and speeds recovery from flu and the common cold
- help counteract hemorrhages caused by anticoagulant drugs
- boosts action of vitamin C
- helps to reduce joint inflammation found in arthritis
- may be useful in preventing cataracts
- works to minimize symptoms of oral herpes
- may work to lower cholesterol levels

Natural Sources

Citrus fruits (primarily the white skin and the segment membranes), apricots, blackberries, cherries, grapes, plums, rose hips, black currants, prunes, spinach, green peppers, rose hips and buckwheat

Deficiencies

Bleeding gums/loose teeth, depression/malaise/tiredness, easy bruising, impaired wound healing, irritability, joint pain, anemia, loss of hair, depression, frequent colds, gallstones, thrombosis, bladder cancer, allergies, hayfever, bedsores, hemorrhaging and bruising, rheumatism, hemorrhoids, rheumatic fever

PABA

PABA is short for *para-aminobenzoic acid* and is necessary for the production of folic acid in the human body. It also helps the body utilize pantothenic acid. It is considered an antioxidant that acts as a coenzyme in the metabolism and assimilation of protein. PABA is commonly found in sunscreens because of its capability to protect against sunburn and the formation of skin cancer.

There is some speculation that supplementing the diet with PABA may restore grey hair to its original color. Laboratory tests for the maintenance of healthy intestines by enhancing intestinal flora activity. It has also been found to have anti-aging properties. Taking sulfa drugs may cause a deficiency of PABA. In addition, ingesting coffee, alcohol and excess water can use up PABA stores.

PABA helps the body make folic acid and use pantothenic acid (vitamin B5). It is destroyed by some antibiotics and sulfa drugs, so PABA intake should be increased while taking those medications.

Benefits

- helps prevent eczema
- aids in healing and relieving pain of burns
- keeps skin healthy and helps prevent wrinkles
- prevents sunburn when applied directly to the skin
- helps restore natural hair color
- plays a role in the production of folic acid
- enhances intestinal flora activity
- may play a role in treating infertility

Natural Sources

Organ meats (liver, kidneys), yeast, molasses, whole grains, wheat, bran

Deficiencies

Gastro-intestinal disorders, fatigue, irritability, depression, headaches, graying hair, Lupus Erythematosis, scleroderma, constipation, irritability

VITAMIN T

Very little research has been done for this vitamin. It is believed that vitamin T assists in the formation of blood platelets which promotes the proper clotting of the blood. In addition, vitamin T may help to improve failing memory and the inability to concentrate. No RDA has been established and there are no supplements for the public on the market.

Benefits

- helps blood coagulation
- prevents some kinds of anemia and hemophilia
- may help improve failing memory and poor concentration

Natural Sources

Egg yolks, sesame seeds, tahini

VITAMIN U

Little is known about this vitamin. It was recently discovered and has yet to be thoroughly researched. Vitamin U is high in chlorophyll which is considered a highly effective natural medicine. Supplies of vitamin U are depleted if exposed to high heat. The Russians have said that the use of vitamin U will cure stomach ulcers.

Benefits

- helps heal ulcers (peptic and duodenal ulcers)

Natural Sources

Raw cabbage, sauerkraut, and celery juice

Minerals

Minerals are necessary to regulate body functions and to maintain tissues. Minerals, as well as vitamins, must be supplied daily either in the diet or through supplements. Minerals are necessary for the body to be able to use vitamins. Minerals are the spark plugs of vitamin use. You can see that this chain of digestive chemical reactions is complicated and interrelated. Without vitamins and minerals you could eat everything in sight and still be malnourished. To complicate things further, minerals cannot be used by the body unless they have been broken down into a digestible form. This process is called chelation, and it frequently costs you up to half the amount of minerals you take. Because of this, it is both cheaper and wiser to purchase mineral supplements in chelated form.

Cutting this one step out of the work your body has to do to use the fuel you need makes a big difference in the effectiveness of the nutritional process. Research done in Poland has shown that vitamins and minerals put in a base of herbs will raise the body's ability to use those vitamins and minerals four-to-five times better than it would be able to without the herbs. This is a form of natural chelation; any vitamin and mineral product assembled this way is naturally chelated.

Many people think that all minerals are the same. We know that there are such things as organic and inorganic minerals. The latter being found int eh soil, but not in as great an abundance as we would like it to be in this twentieth century. Our soil has been leached by wind and rain and over-farming. The farm bureau recommends that certain elements be put back and these are the elements that make it grow red, green, brown and fast. Because of this type of farming, the foods that we think are so good for us really have little taste and is a lot smaller portion of the nutrients that we need and should have. Once they have harvested the crops, the handling of the crop and many times long term cold storage depletes more of the nutrients from the plant. Many people think that we can use inorganic minerals for our mineral needs. In truth, we may be able only to absorb 9 to 19 percent of those minerals and the 19 percent if they have been chelated.

The body loves and wants to have natural and organic minerals and the minerals when they are in a colloidal state, can have up to 95 percent absorption. This is called efficiency and is the way the good Lord intended. Some people don't know or don't understand that we can take vitamins till they run back out of our nose, they won't do a thing without minerals. Minerals are the activators of the vitamins. Colloidal minerals are microscopic and have a negative electrical charge. Colloidal minerals are considered to be non-toxic and when taken in liquid form, this many times increases the absorption factor.

Vitamins are organic. That is, they are built of chemical structures based on carbon. But minerals are not basically carbons (with the exception of a few organic irons). Just the right combinations of vitamins and minerals are very important. Keep the following guidelines in mind as you plan your balanced diet.

BORON

Boron was first discovered in 1910, but it was not until approximately 1982 that is was found to be essential to good health in humans. A number of studies around the world where the soil is deficient in boron seem to develop osteoarthritis more quickly. It seems to help with pain and the stiffness of arthritis and is needed to build and maintain healthy cell membranes along with bones. A combination of calcium, magnesium, vitamin D and the trace mineral boron may help prevent osteoporosis.

Natural Sources

Apples, grapes, grape juice, vegetables, fruits, nuts cider and raisin

Deficiences

Osteoporosis, arthritis, poor bone development, stunted growth

CALCIUM

Calcium is a mineral that is crucial in the proper formation of strong bones and teeth. It also plays a vital role in maintaining regular heartbeat and the proper transmission of nerve impulses. Calcium stores determine the effect peristaltic action of the intestines and the health of muscle fiber. For this reason, muscle cramps can result if calcium is lacking. This mineral is also necessary for blood clotting and is believed to help prevent the development of colon cancer.

Recent studies have shown that calcium may also help to reduce high blood pressure and can minimize bone loss that commonly occurs to post-menopausal women resulting in osteoporosis. In addition, the presence of calcium can help protect the bones and teeth from lead toxicity. In children who have a low calcium level and are exposed to lead, absorption of the lead is much higher. Calcium also works to regulate the acid-alkaline balance in the blood, metabolizes iron and can help protect against radiation exposure. Calcium and phosphorus should be balanced two-to-one in the human body.

Vitamin D is necessary for proper use of calcium. Growing children and hypoglycemics benefit from increased calcium intake. A deficiency of calcium can result in the following symptoms: muscle cramps, brittle nails and bones, nervousness, heart palpitations, eczema, hypertension, tooth decay and insomnia. Ingesting aspirin, chocolate, mineral oil, excess animal protein, salt and phosphorus can deplete calcium supplies in the body.

Benefits

- prevents rickets
- promotes growth and maintenance of healthy teeth and bones
- maintains cardiovascular system, including regulating heart beat
- supports nervous system, particularly transmission of nerve impulses, calms nerves
- increases a person's ability to withstand pain
- relieves muscle spasms
- relieves menstrual cramps
- helps treat insomnia
- eases "growing pains"
- nothing heals without enough calcium
- helps to prevent and reverse osteoporosis
- protects the body against exposure to lead and radiation

- may reduce the risk of colon cancer
- helps with retarded growth and osteomalacia

Natural Sources

Dairy products, peanuts, sunflower seeds, walnuts, soybeans, dried beans, wheat germ, almonds, green leafy vegetabls, salmon, sardines, carob, barley, blackstrap molasses, dandelion greens, dulse, prunes, tofu and whey, yogurt, bonemeal, sesame, legumes, shellfish, nuts, seaweeds

Deficiencies

Bone diseases, teeth and gum disease, menstrual cramps, arthritis, bone spurs, brittle fingernails, cognitive impairment, delusions, depression, eczema, hyperactivity, hypertension, insomnia, irritability, limb numbness, muscle cramps, nervousness, neuromuscular excitability osteomalacia, osteoporosis, palpitations, periodontal disease, pica (eating lead paint), ricketa, retarded growth, tetany, tooth decay, leg cramps, excessive and long menstruation

CHLORINE

Organic chlorine participates in the production of gastric juices which help to facilitate proper digestion. In addition, it works to regulate heart action and normalize blood pressure. Chlorine also contributes to the process of expelling waste from the body and in so doing helps to purify the blood. It boosts liver action and promotes healthy, skin, teeth and bones. It also plays a role in keeping the acid/alkaline balance of the blood in check. Some studies have shown that natural chlorine also assists the immune system by fighting bacterial and viral infections. Ingesting high amounts of table salt can create an excess of inorganic chlorine. Too much chlorine may destroy vitamin E stores and intestinal flora.

Most people who eat an average amount of sea salt each day get adequate chlorine.

Those whose water is chlorinated should eat yogurt to restore intestinal bacteria. They should also increase their intake of vitamin C and vitamin E.

Benefits

- promotes healthy teeth and hair
- aids digestion
- may help control colic
- helps to boost a sluggish liver
- works to treat skin rashes and other skin disorders
- helps the body heal tissue injuries

Natural Sources

Sea salt, (sodium/chloride) olives, seaweed, fish, raw goat's milk, raw cheeses, sardines, and rye flour

Deficiencies

Loss of hair and teeth, difficult digestion, poor muscle contractability

CHROMIUM

Chromium is a mineral that plays a vital role in the metabolism of glucose or sugar in the body. It activates several enzymes that are necessary for this process to occur. Chromium also contributes to the synthesis of cholesterol, fats and proteins. It is the major mineral involved in insulin production and for this reason is believed to substantially augment the body's ability to regulate blood sugar levels. Not surprisingly, a lack of chromium interferes with efficient insulin production and utilization. Some studies even suggest that disorders like diabetes and hypoglycemia may be, in actuality, chromium deficiencies. Chromium picolinate or Chromium nicotinate (niacin bound chromium) are considered the best form of this mineral for its excellent glucose lowering properties. When Chromium and Vanadium are used together the need for insulin replacement is greatly lowered. It is estimated that as high as 95 percent of all diabetics have a deficiency in chromium.

Because of the intrinsic relationship between blood sugar and the metabolism of fats, chromium can also help to lower cholesterol levels.

Low plasma chromium levels are sometimes an indication of coronary artery disease. Ongoing research indicates that chromium may also increase lean body mass while reducing the percentage of body fat.

The average American diet is believed to be chromium deficient. There is a widespread lack of this mineral in soil and water supplies. In addition, the typical American diet, which is high in refined white sugar, flour and fats, further depletes chromium supplies in the body. Strenuous running and other stressful athletic activities may also increase the body's requirement of chromium.

Benefits

- helps prevent diabetes
- deters arteriosclerosis
- aids growth
- helps prevent and correct high blood pressure
- works to lower blood cholesterol levels
- may increase lean body mass and reduce body fat
- may prevent tendencies toward hypoglycemia

Natural Sources

Meat, shellfish, wheat germ, rye, green peppers, clams, chicken, corn oil, Brewer's yeast, brown rice, cheese, whole grains, sugar beets, black strap molasses and calf's liver

Deficiencies

Anxiety, fatigue, hypoglycemia, diabetes, retarded growth/short life span, hypercholesterolemia (high blood cholesterol), atherosclerosis, glucose intolerance

COBALT

Cobalt is a mineral that plays an important role in assisting the body's ability to assimilate and synthesize vitamin B12. In addition, it also stimulates the production of enzymes required for a variety of body processes. Cobalt also participates in the production of red blood cells as well as facilitates cell maintenance. The presence of cobalt also boosts the ability of cells to assimilate iron. Cobalt cannot be made in the body and must be supplied by the diet. Ingesting alcohol, some sleeping pills, and estrogen can deplete cobalt supplies. In addition, an overexposure to sunlight can also destroy cobalt.

Benefits

- helps prevent anemia
- builds red blood cells
- may decrease nervousness
- is considered a growth booster
- may be useful in regulating heart palpitations

Natural Sources

Meat, kidney, liver, fruits, poultry, clams, oysters, green leafy vegetables, buckwheat, figs, oysters, dairy products, apricots and sea vegetation

Deficienies

Pernicious anemia, retarded growth rat

COPPER

Copper is found in virtually all body tissues including the hair. Copper helps the body to absorb and utilize iron and also participates in the formation of bone, hemoglobin and red blood cells. It works with zinc and vitamin C to form elastin, an important constituent of skin and bone integrity. Copper is required for the ability to taste properly. In addition, it is involved in the healing process, energy production and hair and skin coloring. Copper participates in the formation of myelin which is the protective covering of the nerves, and it also helps to maintain muscle tone and boost the immune system.

Interestingly, abnormally high levels of copper have been found in individuals suffering from viral infections, rheumatoid arthritis, rheumatic fever, lupus and heart attack.

One of the earliest signs of a copper deficiency is the development of osteoporosis due to the vital role that copper plays in collagen formation in the bones.

Most people who eat balanced diets get adequate copper. Supplementary copper is rarely prescribed and care should be taken not to over-treat oneself with it. Excessive amounts of copper can keep you awake at night, cause irregular menstrual periods, bring on depression, or increase hair loss. JR copper is required for the body to make proper use of iron, vitamin C and zinc.

Benefits

- maintain high energy level
- helps prevent anemia and edema
- may help to prevent osteoporosis
- may be useful in the treatment of leukemia
- helps to treat bedsores

Natural Sources

Whole wheat, nuts, liver, avocados, whole wheat, dried beans, peas, liver, shrimp, most seafood, prunes, almonds, green leafy vegetables, blackstrap molasses, organ meats and bonemeal, seaweeds, soybeans, raisins, blueberry, legumes, whole grains

Deficiencies

Blood vascular defects, anemia, impaired respiration, skin lesions, bone disease, loss of sense of taste, loss of hair color, infantile diarrhea, depression, fragile bones/arthritis, hypercholesterolemia (high blood cholesterol), otosis (lipping of epiphyseal plates), edema, stomach ulcers, aneurysm/cerebral hemorrhage, criminal behavior, retarded growth, pernicious anemia, weakness, poor iron utilization

FLUORINE

Synthetic fluorine is a toxic poison that is sometimes found in water, vitamins, and toothpaste. Natural fluorine is beneficial to the body. An excess of either natural or synthetic fluorine can cause mottling or discoloration to the teeth. Fluorine is an essential trace mineral concentrated in the teeth and bones. It helps the body use calcium. Fluorine and sodium are two elements that enable the body to more efficiently utilize calcium. Fluorine is called the decay resistant element and because of its relationship with calcium, can help to prevent spine curvature and other bone deformities. Fluorine has also been found to reduce the acid content of the mouth which helps to ward off tooth decay.

For years controversy has raged over whether water should be artificially fluoridated. Proponents of fluoridation have argued that its addition would promote healthier bones and teeth and less tooth decay. Opponents contend that toxic levels of fluorine, from which fluoride is derived could build up in the body and cause toxicity, which could damage the immune system. In more than half the cities in the U.S. fluoridation has become the rule rather than the exception. Inorganic fluorine, unlike natural fluorine is considered to be a highly poisonous substance. Exposure to heat, and ingesting refined foods, sugar, aluminum and fluoride salts can impair the body's ability to absorb naturally occurring fluorine. It has been read in the records of Congress, the studies showing that artificial fluoride whether in water or in toothpaste to be one of the causes of cancer in the human body. Dr. John Yiamouylannis in his book, *Fluoride, The Aging Factor,* estimates that 30 to 50,000 die each year because of consumption of fluoridation. He and Dr. Burk, formerly chief chemist at the National Cancer Institute have done an enormous job in documenting their research in this area.

Benefits

- strengthens bones
- builds resistance to tooth decay
- boost the immune system in fighting viral infections
- may help to decrease hair loss

- has a beneficial effect on eye disorders
- may contribute to lowering the risk of osteoporosis
- works to facilitate the utilization of calcium

Natural Sources

Seafoods, gelatin, salmon, wheat germ, liver, whole wheat, garlic, beets, lettuce, cabbage, radishes, egg whites, raw goat's milk, avocados, brown rice and oats

Deficiencies

Excessive levels may increase the incidence of Mongolism, dental caries, osteoporosis

IODINE

Approximately three quarters of the body's supply of iodine is found in the thyroid gland. While iodine is needed only in trace amounts, it is vital to maintain thyroid gland health and function. It enables the thyroid to regulate body metabolism which influence physical and mental growth, affecting all nerves, muscles, circulation and cell processes. Iodine also plays a significant role in regulating cholesterol levels, and in preventing anemia. It is vital for a healthy lymphatic system and is believed to protect the brain against some toxins. The use of iodine to protect against radiation exposure is also being researched. In addition, in China the link between hearing loss in children and iodine deficiency is currently under investigation.

The classic iodine deficiency disease is goiter, in which the thyroid gland becomes enormously enlarged. The use of iodized salt has greatly decreased the incidence of goiter. Mental retardation may occur from a lack of iodine in children. Recently, an iodine deficiency has been linked to breast cancer.

Some foods actually block the uptake of iodine into the thyroid gland when eaten in large quantities. These include: peaches, rutabagas, strawberries, cabbage, peanuts, spinach and radishes. Too much iodine in the diet will produce a metallic taste, mouth sores, vomiting and swollen salivary glands.

Sufficient iodine for most people is supplied in regular multivitamin and mineral tablets. Those who live in regions where the soil is iodine-poor (the Midwest, for example) and women who are pregnant or nursing might need more.

Benefits

- helps prevent goiter and hypothyroidism
- encourages growth
- boosts energy level
- helps system burn excess fat
- aids in maintaining mental alertness and the ability to think quickly
- promotes healthy hair, skin, teeth, and nails
- promotes healthy tonsils, which are part of the lymphatic and immune system
- may help protect the thyroid gland from radiation exposure
- may play a role in treating obesity
- helps to regulate irregular heartbeat due to metabolism imbalances
- may contribute to lowering cholesterol levels
- can help to prevent cretinism in newborns

Natural Sources

Seafood, spinach, carrots, pears, tomatoes, pineapple, watercress, vegetables, grown in iodine rich soil, particularly garlic, onions, eggplant, mushrooms and potatoes, wheat germ, sea salt, seaweeds, fish, fish liver oil, mushroom

Deficiencies

Goiter, obesity, irritability, cold extremities, dry hair, fatigue, hypothyroidism, low basal body temperature, brittle nails, physical and mental impairment, nervousness, headaches, metabolic disturbances, malaise, constipation

IRON

The most important function of iron is the intrinsic role it plays in the production of hemoglobin in the red blood cells of the body.

Seventy-Five percent of all the iron in the human body is located in the hemoglobin of red blood cells. Hemoglobin is responsible for carrying oxygen from the lungs to all other body cells and tissues. Iron is also essential for the synthesis of numerous enzymes and is vital for proper growth and resistance to disease and infection. For this reason, iron is considered crucial to a healthy immune system and plays an invaluable role in energy production.

In addition, iron improves circulation, intensifies mental vitality and boosts liver and kidney functions. The proper oxygenation of cells is profound in its implication and can promote vigor, youth and overall health.

Recent studies have shown that iron utilization is impaired by the presence of rheumatoid arthritis and cancer, resulting in the subsequent development of anemia. A significant iron deficiency has also been found in people suffering from candidiasis and chronic herpes infections.

Iron deficiency symptoms include: brittle nails, hair and nail beds that are ridged or spoon-shaped, hair loss, fatigue, pallor, dizziness and anemia. An excess build-up of iron in the tissues has been associated with a rare disease called hemochromatosis. Ingesting excess phosphates, food additives, caffeine, and too much manganese can cause a depletion of iron.

Iron is necessary for the body to absorb and use B vitamins. In turn, vitamin C and copper, cobalt, and manganese must be present for the body to use iron. Those who should take extra iron include menstruating women and those who drink lots of coffee or tea.

Benefits

- prevents and helps treat anemia
- promotes growth
- builds resistance to disease
- restores healthy skin tone
- guards against fatigue
- may help decrease the risk of herpes and candida
- should be supplemented for those suffering from alcoholism, bleeding ulcers and heavy menstrual periods
- may increase resistance to cold and other viruses

Natural Sources

Red meat, organ meats (liver, kidney, heart), egg yolks, clams, oysters, dried peaches, nuts, beans, asparagus, apricots, fish, wheat germ, oatmeal, almonds, avocados, beets, blackstrap molasses, dates, dulse, lima beans, lentils, millet, pears, dried prunes, raisins, egg yolks, cherries, whole grains, green leafy vegetables, dried fruits, poultry, seaweed, legumes

Deficiencies

Anemia, weakness, pale skin, brittle nails, breathing difficulty, chlorosis, anorexia, confusion, constipation, depression, dizziness, dysphagia, fatigue, GI upset, growth retardation, headaches, ice eating (pica), irritability, palpitations, tachycardia, loss of hair, loss of resistance to infections, impairment of I.Q., irregular heartbeat, inflamed tongue

MAGNESIUM

Along with calcium and phosphorus, magnesium is absolutely essential for the development and maintenance of strong healthy bones. Another of magnesium's vital roles is the part it plays in facilitating nerve function and muscle relaxation. Studies have also confirmed that magnesium stores are linked with susceptibility to depression, dizziness, twitching, heart disease and high blood pressure. In addition, magnesium protects the arteries from stress and plays a part in the formation of bone. Magnesium also works with body enzymes to metabolize sugar which is stored in the liver and provides energy on demand.

Magnesium may also decrease or even prevent the risk of certain complications of pregnancy such as premature labor and an underdeveloped fetus. If taken prior to the menstrual period, it is believed that magnesium can decrease abnormal food cravings and erratic behavior associated with PMS.

Magnesium is essential for the body to be able to use calcium and vitamin C. It helps convert blood sugar into usable energy. Women who take birth control pills and anyone who drinks alcohol should increase their magnesium. Since magnesium neutralizes stomach acids, it should not be taken directly after a meal.

Although magnesium is widely distributed in foods many groups of people are at risk for developing deficiencies. Alcoholics, diabetics and anyone taking cyclosporin A or diuretics may be susceptible. People with gastrointestinal disorders and those who live highly stressful lives may also suffer from a lack of magnesium. It has been claimed that a deficiency of magnesium is the number two cause of heart death in the United States. It has been shown to keep calcium in solution thus preventing calcium from causing plaquing in the arteries, stones and spurs, thus making calcium available for maintenance and repair in the body. Lack of magnesium cause the bowels to lock up and menstrual cramps. Magnesium is nature's relaxer and thus prevents muscle spasms, heart seizure, muscle cramps, menstrual cramps, and constipation. It makes life easier and smoother. Hosptials are now using magnesium for angina pains which is more effective than beta-blockers. It is also being used in the hospitals as a laxative in place of the toxic chemical laxatives they were using.

Benefits

- Helps prevent heart attack and keeps the cardiovascular system healthy
- relieves indigestion
- aids in resisting depression
- helps prevent calcium deposits and kidney and gall stones
- improves dental health
- relaxes muscle
- may help to prevent premature birth
- supplies energy by metabolizing sugar stored in the liver
- enables calcium to be assimilated
- may help to alleviate some symptoms of PMS

Natural Sources

Yellow corn, dark green vegetables, lemons, grapefruit, figs, nuts, seeds, apples, dairy products, blackstrap molasses, brown rice, figs, garlic, kelp, millet, salmon, tofu, torula, whole grains, seaweeds, legumes, sesame, green leafy vegetables, fish

Deficiencies

Muscular excitability, confusion, kidney stones, tooth decay, exhaustion, fast heart beat, convulsions, anxiety, irritability, restlessness, birth soft bones, kidney stones, confusion, birth defects, hypothermia, insomnia, muscle pain and weakness, SIDS, seizures, heart attacks, nervousness, depression, tremors, noise sensitivity, hyperactivity, neuromuscle irritability, tachycardia

MANGANESE

Manganese is a trace mineral that functions in minute quantities in the body. It is required for the breakdown of protein and fats and is involved in bone growth and development. Manganese is also vital for the proper functioning and health of the nerves and may decrease the incidence of epileptic seizures. Manganese is also essential for iron-deficient anemics and is required for the utilization of thiamine and vitamin E. Manganese contributes to the production of mother's milk and is a key element in the production of the enzymes which oxidize fats and metabolize purines.

Some experiments indicate that a deficiency of manganese may play a role in the ability to tolerate glucose. It is also accepted that a lack of manganese has a strong adverse effect on the immune system. The presence of manganese stimulates the production of antibodies, and phagocytes which fight infection and disease.

During pregnancy or at times of dramatic growth, requirements of manganese are greatly increased. In view of the fact that manganese is poorly absorbed and is severely absent from refined foods, many health care practitioners believe that the recommendation for manganese is far too low. Ingesting large amounts of iron, phosphorus or calcium can also deplete manganese stores in the body.

Those who drink a great deal of milk or eat a large amount of meat may need additional manganese.

Benefits

- promotes proper development and function of central nervous system, thyroid hormones, and skeletal and reproductive systems
- required in digestion and metabolism of food
- improves reflexes
- reduces irritability
- eliminates fatigue
- improves memory
- helps to counteract some symptoms of PMS and works to regulate menstrual periods
- may help improve failing eyesight
- may lower the risk of epileptic seizures
- boost the defenses of the immune system
- contributes to glucose tolerance
- considered to be the love element

Natural Sources

Whole-grain cereals, nuts, peas, green leafy vegetables, beets, egg yolks. avocados, seaweed, blueberries, legumes, pineapple, barley, buckwheat, parsley, carrot, celery, liver, bran

Deficiencies

Dizziness, hearing loss, diabetes, paralysis, ataxia, convulsions, glandular disorders, atherosclerosis, hypoglycemia, tinnitus, weak ligaments and muscular coordinations, allergies, epileptic seizures, fatigue, joint problems, pancreatic atrophy, glucose intolerance, hypercholesterolemia

MOLYBDENUM

Molybdenum is required by the body in extremely small amounts for the metabolism of nitrogen. It contributes to the conversion of purines to uric acid and promote normal cell functions. Like so many other minerals, molybdenum is vital to enzyme action involving xanthine oxidase. It is found in the liver, bones, and kidneys and enables iron stored in the liver to be utilized by the body.

Molybdenum also boosts the oxygen carrying capacity of red blood cells and helps to eliminate toxic nitrogen waste. A low intake of this mineral is associated with disorders of the mouth and gums and with the development of cancer. If the diet is high in refined and processed foods or excess copper, a deficiency of molybdenum can occur. A deficiency of molybdenum may cause impotence in older males. Massive intakes of molybdenum may produce gout.

Molybdenum helps the body convert food into usable energy. It also contributes to the utilization of iron.

Benefits

- helps prevent anemia
- helps to prevent certain mouth and gum disorders
- must be present in adequate amounts to prevent male impotence in older men
- modulates calcium/magnesium/copper metabolism

Natural Sources

Dark green leafy vegetables, peas, beans, nuts, whole grains. buckwheat, meats and barley

Deficiencies

Anemia and premature aging, copper deficiency

PHOSPHORUS

Phosphorus is the second most plentiful mineral in the body next to calcium, and like calcium, most of it is located in the bones and teeth. This mineral is intrinsic to the proper bone and tooth development and also contributes to cell growth, the normal contraction of heart muscle and kidney function.

Phosphorus also participates in fat metabolism by combining with fats in the blood to form phospholipids, which comprise the cell membrane. Phosphorus assists he body in utilizing vitamins and helps to convert food to energy. The proper balance of magnesium, calcium and phosphorus is optimal for total health.

A deficiency of phosphorus is rare because it is so readily available in so many foods. A depletion can occur if aluminum-containing antacids are ingested over a long period of time. On the other hand, excess phosphorus consumption is much more common. A diet that is overly rich in phosphorus combined with a low calcium intake may predispose one to developing osteoporosis. A diet that consists of junk foods is notoriously high in phosphorus and low in calcium.

Vitamin D is also necessary for phosphorus to be effective.

Benefits

- prevents rickets and pyorrhea
- builds healthy bones and teeth
- aids regular heartbeat and normal kidney function
- decreases arthritis pain
- promotes general growth and healing of tissues
- helps to regulate blood pressure
- works with calcium and magnesium in the body

Natural Sources

Fish, poultry, meat, eggs, seeds, nuts, whole grains, barley, rice bran, dried fruit, garlic, salmon, legumes, glandular meats, green vegetables, seaweeds

Deficiencies

Anorexia, anxiety, apprehension, bone pain, dyspnea, physical and mental fatigue, irritability, numbness, pica, weakness, weight loss, pyorrhea, dental decay, anemia, nervous disorders, retarded growth, paresthesias, sight changes, tremulousness

POTASSIUM

The cell of the human body contain more potassium than any other mineral. Potassium is essential for the maintenance of fluid within the cells and is necessary for the chemical reactions that take place there. Potassium is also important for a healthy nervous system and works with sodium to keep the proper acid/alkaline balance in the blood. Potassium contributes to a regular heart rhythm and may actually help control high blood pressure.

Potassium deficiency can result in people who are using diuretics and laxatives. In addition, kidney disorders, prolonged vomiting and chronic diarrhea cause potassium to be lost. Because potassium is also needed for normal hormone secretion, excess stress can tax the adrenal glands and also cause potassium to be lost. Using alcohol, and taking cortisone can also deplete potassium stores in the body.

Conditions which may indicate need for additional potassium include hypoglycemia, severe diarrhea, mental or physical stress, long periods of fasting or dieting. The increase of the use of salt as a preservative has increased the need for potassium.

Benefits

- aids in skin's elasticity
- helps keep heart rhythms normal
- aids in regulating body's water balance
- encourages clear thinking
- helps control allergies
- aids in disposal of body wastes
- helps reduce blood pressure
- aids in slowing aging
- helps to combat the effects of physical and mental stress
- may have a calming effect on the nerves
- taking supplements helps to replenish potassium which is lost by taking drugs for high blood pressure

Natural Sources

Citrus fruits, green leafy vegetables, watercress, mint leaves, sunflower seeds, bananas, potatoes, fish, apricots, avocados, figs, dried fruits, garlic, raisins, tourla, squash, almonds and yams

Deficiencies

Depression, constipation, arrhythmia, acne, cognitive impairment, growth retardation, edema, ECG changes, fatigue, glucose intolerance, hypotension, nervousness, palpitations, respiratory distress, muscle weakness, "salt" retention, tachycardia (rapid heart beat), insomnia, high blood cholesterol, low blood sugar, indigestin, flatulence, paralysis

SELENIUM

Selenium is a mineral that is often lacking due to low soil content or faulty eating habits. Selenium is a vital antioxidant, particularly when it is combined with vitamin E. Selenium helps to protect the immune system by preventing the formation of free radicals which can damage human cells. Selenium works with vitamin E to boost the production of antibodies and to facilitate the oxygenation of tissues. In this regard selenium is good in promoting a healthy heart. People who are deficient in selenium have a great risk of developing heart disease.

When combined with vitamin E, selenium may be effective in the treatment or prevention of skin conditions such as acne and seborrheic dermatitis. It is also needed for pancreatic health and tissue elasticity. Danish research has recently found a link between low selenium levels and rheumatoid arthritis. The same correlation was discovered with the incidence of muscular dystrophy.

Because selenium is considered an antioxidant it is considered an anti-cancer mineral which also promotes energy, vigor and stamina. Ingesting high amounts of fat and prolonged stress can deplete selenium supplies. Refining foods and using high cooking temperatures destroys selenium.

In general, men need a little more selenium than women do. Selenium is an antioxidant and thus enhances the immune system.

Benefits

- slows down aging process
- prevents heart disease
- maintains elasticity in tissues
- helps treat and prevent dandruff
- provides protection from certain cancer
- combats harmful metals in our environment
- may help to prevent rheumatoid arthritis
- works to rejuvenate the elderly in terms of alertness and vigor

- may be helpful in treating emphysema
- works well in combination with vitamin E

Natural Sources

Bran, wheat germ, tuna, tomatoes, onions, broccoli, bran, asparagus, mushrooms, brown rice, garlic, liver, salmon, torula and whole grains

Deficiencies

"Heart attack," cancer risk, cystic fibrosis, cataracts, growth retardation, impaired immunity, muscular dystrophy, pancreatic atrophy, livercirrhosis, sterility in males, premature aging, Kwashiorkor disease, heart disease infections

SILICON

Silicon is required for the development of bone and connective tissue. It is involved in the formation of collagen which is vital to healthy nails, skin, and hair. Silicon is necessary to maintain flexibility in the arteries and plays an important role in preventing coronary heart disease.

Silicon works with fluorine and helps the body increase stamina and resistance to disease. It helps to counteract the effects of aluminum and in this regard is believed to help prevent osteoporosis and possible Alzheimer's disease. As the body ages, silicon levels drop, therefore, the elderly need increased amounts of silicon.

Other elements such as boron, calcium, magnesium, manganese and potassium boost the body's ability to utilize silicon. Eating an excess of fats and sugars can deplete silicon supplies in the body. Silicon is found in high concentrations in the hair, skin and nails.

Benefits

- promotes healing
- promotes growth of nails and hair

- stops splitting of nails and hair
- aids in the retention and utilization of calcium
- aids in the retention of B vitamins
- aids in sweating

Natural Sources

Skins of fruits and vegetables, horsetail, gelatin, oats, barley, cereals, rice polishings, alfalfa, beets, bell peppers and soybeans

Deficiencies

Depression, crying spells, sensitivie to noise, hypersensitive, respiratory distrubances, dandruff, dry skin, scabs, scrofula, acne problems, dental caries, inability to think clearly, cataracts, lip sores, gum boils

SODIUM

Sodium has recently gained a bad reputation in dietary circles, however, it is necessary for maintaining the proper water balance and acid/alkaline content of the blood. Sodium is essential for healthy stomach, nerve and muscle function. It is also considered a constituent of the lymphatic system and assists in the elimination of carbon dioxide from the lungs.

Sodium also works with potassium in regulating the transportation of nutrients and waste in and out of the cell membrane. Although a lack of sodium rarely occurs, its symptoms include: low blood sugar, confusion, weakness, dehydration, heart palpitations and lethargy. Getting an excess of sodium is much more common.

Most people eat much more salt than they realize or than they need to eat. It is easier to add sodium to your diet than to eliminate or cut down on it. An excess of sodium may contribute to high blood pressure. It is recommended that most people cut their salt intake. However, for those *few* who need extra salt, kelp is an ideal supplement. The bloodstream is high in sodium while the cells are high in potassium. The exchange of these minerals is called our electrolyte balance. This is done through what is called our sodium-potassium pump. Dr. Corwin West has proven that when the sodium-potassium pump is not working well, we get excessive sodium in the cells; and if this process is not reversed, death is imminent.

Benefits

- prevents sunstroke and heat prostration
- aids in proper function of muscles and nerves
- promotes digestion of carbohydrates
- in some cases helps prevent neuralgia

Natural Sources

Sea salt, shellfish, carrots, beets, artichokes, dried beef, whey, okra and celery, watercress, black mission figs and goat's milk

Deficiencies

Headaches, muscular cramps, weakness, abdominal cramps, anorexia, confusion, crying jags, dizziness, flatulence, fatigue, depression, hypotension, memory loss, lethargy, infections, illusions, nausea and vomiting, taste loss, weight loss, seizures, collapse of blood vessels, loss of appetite, neuralgia

SULFUR

Sulfur is an acid-forming mineral that is part of certain amino acids. It is known as the beauty mineral because it helps to keep the complexion clear and the hair glossy. In addition, it participates in the production of colllagen which prevents skin dryness and promotes elasticity. Sulfur works in combination with B-complex vitamins and acts as an oxidizing agent. It is required for th efficent assimilation of proteins and is involved in promoting normal heart muscle function.

Sulfur helps to purify the blood, resists bacteria and works to protect the protoplasm of human cells. Sulfur also stimulates liver secretions and serves to protect tissues from toxins such as pollutants or radiation exposure. Sulfur is believed to slow the aging process and may possibly extend life span. Exposure to moisture or heat may destroy or inhibit the action of sulfur in the body.

Most people whose diet includes adequate protein are also getting enough sulfur.

Benefits

- Sulfur promotes healthy hair, skin, nails
- applied creams, helps treat various skin problems
- sulfur maintains oxygen balance for proper brain function
- supports the liver in bile secretion
- helps combat bacterial infections
- sulfur works to purify the blood
- may extend life span and delay the aging process
- sulfur helps to protect the body from toxins and radiation

Natural Sources

Beef, fish, eggs, dried beans, cabbage, garlic, kale, onions, soybeans, turnips, wheat germ, chervil, parsley and certain amino acids

Deficiencies

Painful joints, high blood sugar, high blood fat levels, dermatitis, imperfect development of hair and nails

VANADIUM

Vanadium is a mineral that is required for healthy cellular metabolism and for he development of strong bones and teeth. It also participates in the growth and reproduction process and works to inhibit the production of cholesterol. Vanadium contributes to good circulation and plays a role in iron metabolism.

A deficiency of vanadium may be linked to kidney and coronary heart disease. There is also some evidence that a lack of vanadium may impair fertility and increase infant mortality. Vanadium is not absorbed easily. Using tobacco decreases the uptake of vanadium.

Vanadium taken in synthetic form can easily be toxic. Chromium and vanadium in combination is required for the glucose tolerance factor and the production of insulin.

Benefits

- cuts down formation of cholesterol in blood vessels
- helps prevent heart attack
- may help to prevent tooth decay
- may help to prevent kidney disease
- helps with the production of insulin

Natural Sources

Fish, vegetable oils, olives, snap beans, dill, radishes, liver and soybeans

Deficiencies

Diabetes, hypoglycemia, increased cholesterol formation in blood vessels and central nervous system, delayed sexual development and sterility

ZINC

Our bodies contain approximately two to three grams of zinc which is distributed throughout the entire body. The highest amounts of zinc are found in the hair, liver, bone, eyes and prostate gland. While the body contains zinc, there are technically no real storage places for this mineral, consequently, the human body needs to be furnished a continual supply of zinc.

Zinc plays a critical role in the production of RNA and DNA which are required for cell division and growth. Several studies have confirmed that low levels of zinc may be responsible for miscarriages and birth defects. Children who were found low in zinc were usually stunted in growth and had poor appetites. The appetite stimulating properties of zinc have proved useful in treating anorexia nervosa.

Zinc also plays an important role in the healing of wounds and in promoting a healthy immune system. Zinc facilitates the sensitivity of taste and smell and also works to protect the liver from toxins. Zinc contributes to the production of male hormones and is needed for the complete action of B-complex vitamins and vitamin E. Silicon and zinc promote the growth and health of hair.

Taking excessive calcium, antacids, alcohol and oral contraceptives may deplete the body's supply of zinc which must be continually replenished.

Alcoholics, diabetics, and those who take large doses of vitamin B6 need to increase their zinc intake. Those who take extra zinc should also take extra vitamin A.

Benefits

- prevents prostate problems
- helps control cholesterol deposits and so prevents arteriosclerosis
- contributes to the formation of insulin
- aids in healing of wounds, both internal and external
- promotes growth and mental alertness
- restores sense of taste and smell
- helps treat infertility
- eliminates white spots on fingernails
- may help regulate menstrual periods
- combats against impotency
- fights against tinnitus
- helps prevent hearing loss
- helps prevent hair loss
- helps to make fragile nails stronger
- fights against adult acne
- helps to make rough skin smoother
- may help treat anorexia nervosa
- zinc is needed to produce hydrochloric acid

Natural Sources

Eggs, Brewer's yeast, wheat germ, ground mustard, pumpkin seeds, fish, lamb chops, lima beans, oyster, mushrooms, pecans, sardines, soy lecithin, torula and avocados

Deficiences

Retarded growth and fatigue, prolonged healing of wounds, potentiates diabetes, loss of smell and taste, acne, prostate problems, anorexia, white spot on finger nails, malaise, arthritis, alopecia, brittle hair and nails, irritability, sexual immaturity, sterility, paranoia, memory loss, impotence, depression, apathy, birth defects, malabsorption, infertility, chronic infections, lack of hydrochloric acid, hormone deficiencies, anemia, psoriasis, anorexia, amnesia, eczema, fatigue, hypercholesterolemia, lethargy

WATER

Water is often a forgotten element essential to proper health. Most people would benefit by increasing their daily water intake. Thirst is the body's way of telling us that more water is needed. Extra glasses of water taken regularly throughout the day (and not just when one feels thirsty) would help people. Drink plenty of water! An ideal amount would be to drink about one glass of liquid (water) every two hours. For dieters, drink a full glass before each meal. (WATER IN AS PURE A STATE AS POSSIBLE IS PREFERED.)

Benefits

- helps keep all systems functioning
- regulates body temperature
- prevents constipation
- aids in dieting by depressing appetite before meals
- prevents dehydration
- helps the body combat fever, disease, and infection by ridding it of impurities
- prevents the formation of kidney stones
- keeps the digestive tract functioning properly

Natural Sources

Drinking water, juices, fruits, vegetables, reverse osmosis water. Fruits are 90 percent distilled water. Bottled water and filtered water are sometimes questionable as to their source and the effectiveness of longevity of the filter. One of the best ways to get purified water is through the use of reverse osmosis units that can be utilized in the home. Even the pharmaceutical people use reverse osmosis (R.O.) units in the making of drugs and baby formulas. Our astronauts have to reuse all water when in space so all their water is purified through an reverse osmosis unit. The best R.O. units will have a pre-filter, then the R.O. membrane followed by a post filter made of activated charcoal. These are considered to be the best. R.O. units do not remove trace minerals which we desperately need which are depleted from our soils. Through their mechanical action of purifying the water, they many times increase the quantity of oxygen in the water. Oxygen also purifies the water and we can certainly use the extra oxygen in our bloodstreams.

Vitamins and Minerals from Herbal Sources

ALUMINUM
gotu kola, chickweed, pennyroyal, buchu, butcher's broom, mullein, grapevine, devil's claw, thyme, echinacea, blue cohosh, sarsaparilla, uva ursi, cramp bark, althea, ginger, dandelion, kelp, senna, dulse, alfalfa

CALCIUM
valerian, buchu, white oak bark, pau d'arco, kelp, cabbage, nettle, senna, crampbark, plantain, bupleurum, barberry, horsetail, Irish moss, damiana, grapevine, pennyroyal, wood betony, thyme, alfalfa, dulse, parsley, alfalfa

CHLOROPHYLL
alfalfa

CHLORINE
alfalfa, dandelion, kelp, parsley, red raspberry

CHROMIUM
hibiscus, spirulina, gymnema, oatstraw, nettle, red clover, stevia, barley grass, lemon grass, horseradish, peach bark, juniper berry, parthenium, pollen, red clover, damiana, safflower, buchu, ginkgo, catnip, alfalfa

COBALT
golden seal, capsicum, dong quai, pau d'arco, dulse, echinacea, eyebright, wild yam, pollen, devil's claw, ho shou wu, pumpkin seed, sarsaparilla, papaya, yerba santa, nettle, damiana, comfrey, mullein, butcher's broom

COPPER
scullcap, sage, white oak bark, horsetail, yucca, pumpkin seeds, gotu kola, alfalfa

FLUORINE
garlic, alfalfa, lemon grass, licorice

IODINE
dulse, garlic, Irish moss, kelp, sarsaparilla, black walnut, dandelion

IRON
devil's claw, chickweed, mullein, pennyroyal, blue cohosh, butcher's broom, kelp, bilberry, burdock, thyme, barberry, catnip, horsetail, celery, althea, yerba santa, milk thistle, uva ursi, red raspberry, dandelion, alfalfa

LITHIUM
kelp

MAGNESIUM
Irish moss, oatstraw, tumeric, licorice, kelp, nettle, senna, dog grass, elecampane, peppermint, boneset, dulse, white willow, pennyroyal, devil's claw, burdock, chickweed, althea, pumpkin seed, bupleurum, astragalus, Siberian ginseng, alfalfa

MANGANESE
red raspberry, grapevine, bilberry, yerba santa, buchu, catnip, ginger, gotu kola, white oak bark, blue cohosh, lady slipper, wood betony, dog grass, hydrangea, uva ursi, spirulina, mistletoe, chickweed, hibiscus, milk thistle, alfalfa

PHOSPHORUS
blue cohosh, bilberry, pumpkin seed, yerba santa, dog grass, soybean, peppermint, cranberry, yellow dock, asparagus, broccoli, horseradish, milk thistle, Siberian ginseng, buchu, cauliflower, ginkgo, fennel, barley, watercress, alfalfa

POTASSIUM
celery, cabbage, parsley, broccoli, asparagus, cauliflower, horseradish, blessed thistle, barley, hydrangea, sage, bupleurum, catnip, hops, lemon grass, dulse, peppermint, feverfew, carrot, scullcap, alfalfa

SELENIUM
hibiscus, catnip, yerba santa, dog grass, ho shou wu, milk thistle, buch, lemon grass, lady slipper, yarrow, valerian, blue cohosh, barberry, blessed thistle, bayberry, althea, dulse, black cohosh, pumpkin seed, sarsaparilla, alfalfa

SILICON
horsetail, dulse, eyebright, echinacea, golden seal, ginger, dog grass, cornsilk, burdock, butcher's broom, hydrangea, lady slipper, thyme, astragalus, turmeric, oatstraw, licorice, gotu kola, lemon grass, alfalfa

SODIUM
dulse, Irish moss, kelp, rose hips, grapefruit, celery, gotu kola, licorice, parsley, cabbage, oatstraw, pennyroyal, comfrey, carrot, buchu, chamomile, safflowers, barley grass, peppermint, wild yam, alfalfa

SULFUR
alfalfa, burdock, capsicum, eyebright, fennel, garlic, Irish moss, kelp, mullein, nettle, parsley, plantain, raspberry, sage, shepherd's purse, thyme

TIN
dog grass, juniper berries, bilberry, milk thistle, dulse, lady slipper, althea, valerian, Irish moss, nettle, barberry, yarrow, blessed thistle, red clover, yellow dock, licorice, kelp, senna, devil's claw, pennyroyal, alfalfa

ZINC
bilberry, mistletoe, scullcap, buchu, pumpkin seed, capsicum, lady slipper, sage, pennyroyal, wild yam, spirulina, chickweed, echinacea, astragalus, nettle, Irish moss, Siberian ginseng, dulse, elecampane, parthenium, alfalfa

TRACE MINERALS
alfalfa, bee pollen, dulse, kelp, spirulina

Vitamins from Herbal Sources

VITAMIN A/Beta-carotene
spirulina, carrot, gotu kola, cabbage, barley grass, peppermint, senna, yellow dock, uva ursi, parsley, horseradish, alfalfa, chaparral, broccoli, blessed thistle, red raspberry, yerba santa, capsicum, nettle, safflower, dandelion, stevia, eyebright, watercres.

VITAMIN B1 (Thiamine)
spirulina, ephedra, asparagus, gotu kola, fenugreek, barley grass, cauliflower, peppermint, wheat germ flour, senna, acerola fruit, burdock, elecampane, grapevine cabbage, barberry, blue cohosh, sage, yellow dock, bilberry, alfalfa

VITAMIN B2 (Riboflavin)
spirulina, peppermint, senna, barley grass, asparagus, broccoli, horseradish, eyebright, cabbage, alfalfa, parsley, gotu kola, echinacea, cauliflower, ephedra, yellow dock, hops, barberry, blue cohosh, capsicum, watercress

VITAMIN B3 (Niacin)
hops, feverfew, red raspberry, ginkgo, eyebright, slippery elm, asparagus, spirulina, cabbage, chamomile, hydrangea, red clover, black cohosh, peppermint, gotu kola, barley grass, damiana, white willow, alfalfa, mullein

VITAMIN B6 (Pyroxidine)
alfalfa

VITAMIN B12 (Cyanocobalamin)
alfalfa, kelp

VITAMIN B15 (Pangamic acid)
bee pollen, cabbage, dandelion, juniper berries, marshmallow, pumpkin seeds

VITAMIN B17 (Amygealin or Laetrile)
apricot kernels, cabbage, celery, chaparral, flax seed, garlic

VITAMIN B-COMPLEX (Biotin)
alfalfa, bee pollen, cauliflower, Korean ginseng, Siberian ginseng, okra, slippery elm, spirulina

VITAMIN B-COMPLEX (Choline)
bee pollen, cabbage, chamomile, Korean ginseng, licorice, peppermint

VITAMIN B-COMPLEX (Folic Acid)
alfalfa, asparagus, bee pollen, broccoli, cabbage, carrot, cauliflower, comfrey, Korean ginseng, kelp, spirulina, watercress

VITAMIN B-COMPLEX (Inositol)
alfalfa, bee pollen, cabbage, echinacea, garlic, onion, spirulina

VITAMIN C
acerola fruit, broccoli, horseradish, cauliflower, rose hips, aloe vera juice, lemon, senna, papaya, cabbage, oranges, yellow dock, asparagus, red raspberry, barley grass, red clover, onion, lobelia, hops, pumpkin seed, alfalfa, bee pollen, burdock, celery, chickweed, garlic, juniper berries, kelp, parsley, spirulina, watercress

VITAMIN D
alfalfa, bee pollen, carrot, chickweed, comfrey, dandelion, garlic, lemon grass, marshmallow, watercress

VITAMIN E
alfalfa, barley grass, bee pollen, broccoli, carrot, peppermint, spirulina, dandelion, kelp, red raspberry, rose hips, watercress

VITAMIN F (Unsaturated Fatty Acids)
angelica, bee pollen, fennel, garlic, ginger, licorice, parsley, spirulina, St. John's wort

VITAMIN G
alfalfa, capsicum, dandelion, gotu kola, kelp

VITAMIN K (Phylloquinone)
alfalfa, bee pollen, cabbage, carrot, cauliflower, chamomile, comfrey, ginger, kelp, broccoli

VITAMIN P (Bioflavonoids)
dandelion, rose hips, juniper berries, lemon, parsley

VITAMIN T
alfalfa, plantain

VITAMIN U
alfalfa, cabbage

Homeopathy and Bach Flower Remedies

About 1976 we were introduced to Bach Flower Remedies. We wondered about them and, like all facets of health that we have been introduced to, began to check it out and use them ourselves. Well, over the years we have used them to help many people as well as our family!

Dr. Edward Bach

Dr. Bach was a highly respected physician in England in the early 1930s and he became convinced, after many years of research and practice, that many of his patients' illnesses were the direct manifestation of mental and emotional stress. He excelled in many areas of medicine in his 20 years of practice. He was a pathologist, bacteriologist and immunologist.

In 1920, through his research in bacteriology, he concluded that certain strains of bacteria found in the intestinal tract were the primary cause of most chronic illnesses. He then developed a series of vaccines which were highly successful in alleviating a wide variety of chronic disorders. Although many orthodox medical doctors hailed his vaccines as a major medical breakthrough, Dr. Bach was not happy with many of the side effects. Shortly, therefore, he was introduced to the field of homeopathy and found that by preparing the vaccines as homeopathic remedies, the side effects were substantially reduced. They were called the Bach nosodes and proved to be a major step forward and many homeopathic physicians came to regard Dr. Bach as one of the foremost contributors to the field of homeopathy since Samual Hahnemann, its founder.

Dr. Bach found that by treating the personality it was a very important factor in curing of illness. He continued with his research and concluded that disease was the consolidation of mental attitudes, the physical manifestation of various negative states of mind. Dr. Bach rejected all his previous work as not addressing the real issues of health and the cure of disease. He gave up his prosperous Harley Street practice and set out for the Welsh countryside, convinced that the simple plants of the field would provide the essential elements necessary to restore health and vitality.

During the time 1930 to 1936, Dr. Bach discovered 38 flowering trees, plants, and special waters, which were used to treat such negative states of mind as uncertainty, impatience, and fear. One need only to identify the state of mind, mood, or personality type and then pick the appropriate flower remedy to match it. These essences are today known as the *Bach Flower Remedies.*

Dr. Bach used extensive research and found the remedies to be completely safe for use, requiring the smallest dosages to be effective. In addition, it was reported the the Bach Flower Remedies would not interfere with or be affected by any other form of medicine a person might be required to take; if improperly chosen they would, at worst, show a lack of effectiveness; and if taken in overdosage, will do no harm.

There are some modern day practitioners who are experimenting with other flowers as remedies also. They are at this date still trying and proving these new remedies, so Dr. Bach's work goes on in this day and age. One such group is based in California and called the Flower Essence Service. They have come upon many new flowers to be used as an aid to emotional problems.

Be assured that Flower Essences are from a homeopathic origin and are so designed to help the body, not hinder it following the principle of "like cures like."

The list that follows has been designed to help you understand not only the reason we would use the Flower Essences, but the results you would hope to achieve from the use of them.

Flower Essence

Negative Side		Positive Side
Hides problems and worries deep within, sleeplessness. Sometimes resorts to drugs or alcohol to dull mental torture. Hides anxiety, behind cheerfulness.	Agrimony	Laugh at worries that are unimportant, optimist, peacemaker, sense of humor. Faces and works with emotional pain. Works toward obtaining true inner peace.
Feels cut off, without spiritual guidance and protection.	Angelica	Feels protected and guided by spirit, especially during experiences such as birth and death.
Unknown fear, terror, anxiety and even panic without the least reason, dread, hidden fears and nightmares.	Aspen	Fearless, deep faith, feels great joy for life. Has confidence and trust to meet the future. In tune with the spiritual part of life.
Insecure, mistrusts the world with cynicism. Not in tune with Higher Self.	Baby Blue Eyes	Trusts as a child, feels at ease with the world. Feels loved and supported.
Lack of humility; critical; not able to put oneself in another person's place. Passing judgment. Intolerant, demands perfection of others.	Beech	Forgiving; deep understanding of people; tolerant. Accepts people as they are, only seeing the good in every situation and within each person.
Finds self in abusive, addictive or violent relationships.	Black Cohosh	Confronts abusive or threatening situations with courage.
Quiet, timid, docile, submissive, easily imposed upon by others. Wants to please, cannot say no, neglects self.	Centaury	Serves wisely, quietly, unobtrusively, keeps individuality, follows higher dictate of inner self. Recognizes own needs, can say no when necessary, acts from inner strength.
Seeks and follows advice of others against his own good judgment. Talkative, saps vitality of others with questions, doubts self. Does not make own decisions.	Cerato	Quiet assurance, self confident, very intuitive, can judge between right and wrong; trusts in his own intuition.
Fear of losing control of thought or actions, of mental and emotional breakdowns, thoughts of suicide, feelings of desperation, destructive urges, compulsive and obsessive.	Cherry Plum	Calm, quiet courage under pressure; much endurance. Retains equanimity under extreme stress. Has faith and trust and feels guided and protected by a Higher Power.
Makes same mistakes over and over again. Does not learn from experience. Continues to repeat destructive patterns of behavior and/or negative relationships.	Chestnut Bud	Good student; learns from own experiences and examples of others; uses wisdom and understands the lessons to be learned.
Outward flow of love is blocked and turned inward. Is overpossessive of others. Self centered, tries to control others. Uses negative ways of getting attention. Wrapped up in self, demanding.	Chicory	Selfless in care and concern of others; gives without thought of return. Allows others freedom to be themselves.
Avoids difficulties or unpleasantness by withdrawing into own world. Listless, apathetic and inattentive. One who daydreams to escape the present. Enjoys sleeping to avoid facing reality.	Clematis	Lively interest in life; practical idealist. Master of own thoughts.
The mind needs cleansing of that which it dislikes and that which fills it with despair and disgust. Has poor self image, feels unclean, with strong feelings of imperfection.	Crab Apple	Complete control of thoughts, wise, broadminded, can transmute disharmony into harmony. Purity of spirit, accepts the physical world and physical body.

Negative Side		Positive Side
Occasionally feels overwhelmed by responsibilities and scope of work. Feels results of efforts are inadequate, this brings on a state of despondency and exhaustion. Feels tasks are too difficult.	Elm	Self-assurance, confidence. Good leader. Unshakable inner conviction. Helps other people. Serves with joy and has the confidence to complete one's chores.
Negative outlook. Suffers from deep depression and dark melancholia. Easily discouraged, especially after a setback. Feelings of doubt, pessimistic.	Gentian	No thought of failure; no obstacle too great; no task too big. Perseveres, keeps faith to go on despite seeming setbacks.
Suppresses painful, negative memories from the past such as early childhood memories and feelings of pain and trauma about past happenings which now affects the present emotional life.	Golden Ear Drops	Abe to face and release memories from childhood or past experiences. Is in touch with ones own spirituality.
Has lost heart and hope. Feels it is useless to try any more. Has given up. Feelings of despair, hopelessness, is easily discouraged and will resign self, believing nothing more can be done.	Gorse	Positive, deep and abiding faith and hope, certain to overcome all difficulties in the end.
Concerned about self. Filled with problems, difficulties and trivia of the day. Talks rapidly and incessantly. Does not like to be alone. Appears not interested in what others have to say.	Heather	Selfless, understanding; willing to listen; unsparing in efforts to help others. Inner serenity, emotionally self sufficient.
Antidote for hatred. Hatred is absence of love. Hatred breeds insecurity, aggressiveness, jealousy, enby and suspicion. Holly protects us from everthing that is not Universal love. Feels cut off from love.	Holly	Can give without return. Loving, tolerant, happy, rejoice for another's good fortune, feels loved, has compassion for everyone.
No interest in the present, no effort to confront existing difficulties. Body left to struggle in present while mind re-lives the past. One who dwells on past happiness such as ambitions not fulfilled or loved ones now gone. Does not expect to be happy again.	Honeysuckle	Retains lessons of the past, but lets past negative experiences pass out of the mind. Lives fully in the present.
Fatigue in mind many times due to boredom. Doubt of strength or ability to face life or work. Monday Morning Blues. Daily tasks of life seem overwhelming, and feels that there is not enough energy to get things accomplished.	Hornbeam	Certain of own ability and strength. Energetic, enthusiastic and involves oneself in life's task; can take heavy responsibility.
Active nervous person who moves, eats and speaks quickly. Intelligent and intuitive, intolerant, good and efficient in whatever they undertake. Impatient with slower people. Enjoys working at own pace.	Impatiens	Great gentleness and sympathy towards others. Capable, decisive, intuitive, clever, abilities far above average. Tolerant of those who are slower.
Not frightened, but convinced he cannot do as well as others. Expects to fail, no confidence, censors self.	Larch	Willing to plunge into life. Is not discouraged by failure, knows he or she did the best they could. Doesn't know the word "can't". Self confident, unconstrained, creative.
Creates barriers and is unable to reach out to others. Is insecure in social situations.	Mallow	Friendly, personable, warm and open hearted.
Full of fears such as fear of the dark, growing old, heights, illness, loss of job, public speaking, etc. Normally shy, retiring, timid, introverted, phobic, and prone to hide anxieties.	Mimulus	Faces all trials and difficulties with equanimity and humor. Great understanding and courage with confidence to face the challenges of life.
Unable to assert oneself, cannot take a stand for one's beliefs, will withdraw with fear in the face of a challenge.	Mountain Pride	Faces life with strong, positive masculine energy.

Negative Side		Positive Side
State of mind is a black depression, a hopelessness. Despairing melancholia comes suddenly and without any reason. Feelings of gloom, despair, depression, without reason.	Mustard	Unshakable inner security, joy and peace.
Strong physically, can stand great strain. When despair becomes too much-may crack and suffer a nervous breakdown. Not knowing when to quit, inflexible. Will continue on even in the face of lost cause, illness or hardship. Strong toiler whom others depend on.	Oak	Brave, fighting against great difficulties without loss of hope or slackening of effort. Courage, stability under all conditions, knows one's limits and when to quit. Well balanced.
Fatigue is total; mind and body are drained of strength and there is absolute exhaustion. Depends too much on physical body for life-expression. No enjoyment in life and feels everything is an effort.	Olive	Patient and long-suffering, showing interest in life. Mind is at peace and finds satisfaction in life.
Self-condemnation, never content with achievements, blames self for not doing better and for mistakes of others. Is critical of self, feels guilty without cause, perfectionist.	Pine	Will take responsibility and burdens of others if necessary. Will acknowledge mistakes but not dwell on them. Has great perseverance and humility. Accepts self, able to forgive self and can release the past.
Fear for others, especially family and those dear to them. Always fearing the worst, obsessive fear and anticipating misfortune or problems for others.	Red Chestnut	Sends out thoughts of safety, health or courage to those who need them. Remains calm, mentally and physically, during emergency. Retains an inner peace and trusts in life's unfoldment.
Feelings of great alarm or terror, deep fear, panic because of illness or fear of death or annihilation, an accident, or emergency.	Rock Rose	Courageous, forgetful of self, inner peace and tranquillity, when facing great challenges. Will risk life to help others.
Hard masters on themselves; strict in their way of living. Practices self-denial and self-martyrdom. Sets rigid standards for self. Puritanism. Denies pleasures in order to set examples for others.	Rock Water	Will forsake original theories and beliefs for higher and better truth. Can forgive themselves and others. Experiences joy and peace in life. Has great flexibility, in touch with emotions.
Unable to accept emotions, fears deep feelings, cannot remove issues of power or anger.	Scarlet Monkeyflower	Faces emotions honestly, communicates directly and clearly.
Suffers from indecision, confused, mood swings. Swayed between two things or possibilities. Experiences extremes of joy or sadness, energy or apathy, pessimism or optimism, laughing or crying.	Scleranthus	Calmness and determination. Quick to make a decision and prompt in action. Poise and balance at all times with the certainty of inner knowing.
Always use in case of an accident, sudden sad news, a bad fright or grievous disappointment. These cause shock as well as unhappiness. Feels great distress, trauma, grief. Refuses to be calmed.	Star of Bethlehem	The comforter and soother of pains and sorrows. If the shock is neutralized, recuperation is accelerated.
Unable to obtain inner peace, feels cut off. Cannot pray or meditate for feeling of contentment.	Star Tulip (Cat's Ears)	Meditates, listens to inner self and others.
Mental torture in the extreme. Terrible, appalling mental despair. The very soul itself seems to be suffering destruction. Feels like cannot go on.	Sweet Chestnut	The kind of faith that can cause miracles. Desire to help others in despair. Shows deep spiritual strength.
Listless, procrastinates, habits that inhibit one's self-purpose in life.	Tansy	Set goals and is deliberate in action, directs oneself.

Negative Side		Positive Side
Over-enthusiasm, over-effort, stress and tension. Holds strong opinions and ideas which hardly ever change and which they wish to impose on others. Fanatic, can be overbearing, strong opinions. Feels the need to convert others to their beliefs.	Vervain	Calm, wise, knows own mind. Allows others the right to opinions. Open-minded, listens to others. It is by being rather than doing that great things are accomplished. Enthusiastic, idealistic, the ability to draw people to them.
Think they know better than anyone else; force their will upon one and all. Demand obedience. Crave power. Can be tyrannical, aggressive and domineering. Natural born leaders, capable.	Vine	Wise, loving, does not dominate, unshakable confidence and certainty. Tolerance for other's individuality and tries to help others to know themselves.
For advancing stages: teething, puberty, change-of-life. Big decisions made during life, such as change of occupation, stepping forward in life, leaving old limits and restrictions. Is overly influenced by other's ideas. Needs to be protected from outside influences and help in adjusting to new situations.	Walnut	Constancy and determination. Carries out beliefs and life's work unaffected by adverse circumstances or unhindered by either the opinions or the ridicule of others. Freedom to follow one's own path in life.
Feel superior to others, and sometimes they are disdainful and condescending. Pride and mental rigidity often manifest themselves in the body as physical stiffness and tension. Remains aloof, withdrawn, has difficulty with social relationships. Loners making it difficult for others to approach and befriend, proud, aloof.	Water Violet	Tranquil; gentle; sympathetic. Have poise, dignity and pass gracefully through life. Values one's social relationships and shares one's talents with others.
Worry or some depressing happening preys upon the mind. Arguments or words that they think should have been said go round and round in the mind. Mind continually working with unwanted thoughts and mental arguments which causes sleeplessness.	White Chestnut	Inner quiet, calm, controls thoughts and imagination, clarity of mind; at peace within and with the world.
Undecided what to do. Delay in finding life's work. So many ideas and ambitions that they cannot come to a decision. Confused and indecisive about direction, trying many activities but never satisfied. Frustration due to determining causes for dissatisfaction.	Wild Oat	Definite ambitions and goals in life. Allows nothing to interfere with purpose. Life filled with usefulness and happiness.
They become resigned. Feel they have to live with it, fatalistic. Does not understand that conditions in life can be changed or eliminated by their own hands and makes no effort to find joy. Takes life as it comes.	Wild Rose	Lively interest in all happenings, enjoys friends, happiness and good health. Finds joy in life and the will to live is strong.
Look upon life with bitterness. Blames everyone but themselves for their misfortunes. Believes their treatment is unjust. Jealous of their fellow man. Feels life is unfair, resentment, is bitter and dwells in self pity.	Willow	Great opinion and faith, sense of humor, see things in right proportion. Forgiveness, kindness, accepts oneself. Takes responsibility for one's self.
Constricts feelings, mainly in chest. Represses emotions, melancholic, holds grief inside.	Yerba Santa	Free-flowing emotion, ability to harmonize breathing with feeling, capable of a full range of human emotion, is able to feel pain and unhappiness.
Use in case of sorrow, sudden bad news, after an accident, shock, fear, terror, panic, any stress or strain. Steadies emotional upsets that are experienced everyday.	Rescue Remedy #39	Cherry Plum, Clematis, Impatiens, Rock Rose and Star of Bethlehem. "ALWAYS HAVE THE RESCUE ESSENCE ON HAND. THE LIFE YOU SAVE MY BE YOUR OWN."

Homeopathy

The name Homeopathy was given to us by Dr. Samuel Hahnemann. He used the Greek words meaning "similar" and "suffering." Dr. Hanemann was a very famous German physician in the 1800s who gave up his medical practice, as he was very disillusioned with what he called modern medical science. He found his patients thought he was almost God, as he could suppress the pain and the symptoms of disease and people thought they were well. But as he said, they would come back with a new problem which he concluded was caused by the suppression of the original disease in the body. He concluded that symptoms should not be suppressed, as they were the patient's body working to overcome the original problem.

Dr. Hahnemann decided when he was retired to do research and write. In his studies in the old text talking about what physicians did to heal, he found such original physicians as Hypocrites, around 400 B.C., along with Paracelsus back in the 1400s and 1550s used different methods than modern science was using. He found that in the ancient books, it talked about using the natural law of similars, and he goes to credit the statement "let likes be cured by likes." He found that if he was using a substance, that if given to a person who did not have the disease, it would create the symptoms of the disease. He found also by diluting down the substance and by shaking it well, that he could use this substance in its diluted form with the person who had the disease and the body would heal itself. He finally acquired many volunteers and would use them in the process he called "proving" and developed many remedies for many problems. He recorded the many symptoms that people developed in the provings and the books are available today called Repertory Homeopathics.

Similar books have been written by some of his disciples such as Kent. Dr. Hanemann had an opportunity to prove his theories during the 1830s cholera epidemics in Europe. He took medications that would create cholera-like symptoms in individuals who did not have cholera, again it was called a "proving." His success rate was that his patients death rate was less than 20 percent when his medical colleagues was well over 50 percent. In Britain, the physician for the Queen of England is an HMD (Homeopathic Medical Doctor) and has been in the family royalty for over 150 years. In fact, the Queen of England supports two hospitals in London that are exclusively homeopathic. Forty percent of doctors that practice in Europe are HMDs. Homeopathy is used especially in Germany, France, Brazil, Argentina and Mexico.

Seventy percent of all the doctors who practice in India are HMDs. It's recorded in history that in the U.S., it was especially successful in the 1849 cholera and the 1878 yellow fever epidemics. That is one of the reasons that scarlet fever and typhoid was brought under control in the U.S. also. At one time, there was as many as 20 colleges teaching homeopathic medicine here in the U.S. The AMA established itself in 1846 and their bylaws say that one of the reasons they formed was to destroy homeopathic medicine and would not even allow homeopathic doctors to become members.

By the late 1800s, the Rockefellers had firmly established themselves as drug producing drug companies. The AMA was becoming very strong at this time influencing state licensing boards, where they could refuse licenses to Homeopaths and forced homeopathic colleges to close. There is still a U. S. Pharmacology of Homeopathy and homeopathic remedies are recognized by the Food and Drug Administration as over-the-counter medications. Even specific therapeutic claims can be made on the bottles. Homeopathics can be compared to the electrical system of a car, but without the gas tank and fuel in the gas tank, the car isn't going to run. Without the fuel in the body called nutrition, our body will not run. When homeopathics are added to nutrition, things work faster, smoother and more efficient and healing is generally more complete.

There are over 2,000 homeopathic medications that the medical doctor, acupuncturist, dentist, chiropractor, and even a veterinarian are using very effectively today. Even lay people are now educating themselves on Homeopathic remedies as they are non-toxic and have no terrible side effects. In fact, there have never been homeopathic remedies ever taken off the market in the approximately 200 years that homeopathics has been used for toxicity. There has never been a homeopathic remedy recalled and taken off the market, but we can't say that about the drug companies and their allopathic medicines. In fact, in the *Physicians Desk Reference* used by the medical doctor for his study of drugs, it said that there has never been a drug medication ever developed that there are not side effects and after effects, some of them very deadly and destructive to the body. Don't forget to read about the Bach Flower Remedies, which are about the physical emotions as these are homeopathic remedies also.

HOW TO USE HOMEOPATHIC REMEDIES

- Homeopathic remedies can be taken topically and internally as well.
- In some cases, especially with the Bach Flower Remedies, they are applied on the pulse points such as on the wrists or on the forehead.
- When taken internally, they can be taken in a milk lactose tablet or a liquid solution with alcohol.
- Generally, there is approximately 15 to 20 drops used internally or three to four drops when used on the pulse.
- Topically, they are used more for emotions.
- When we use more than one homeopathic remedy at a time, they should be taken alone, so we should separate those remedies 15 to 20 minutes apart.
- Generally, they are taken about a half hour before eating or after eating.
- Try to not take them with food. If taken with foods, they will be beneficial but not as effective.
- Be aware that we are using the vibratory frequencies of these diluted products in order to make changes in the body. You also need to be aware that anything with caffeine, it can knock out up to 85 percent effectiveness of some homeopathic products.
- Another 10 percent can be effected by volatile oils such as peppermint oil, tei fu oil, eucalyptus oil, etc.
- When taken orally, it should be placed under the tongue in either liquid or tablets and hold for up to 20 seconds before swallowing.

CANDIDA

Fungus cannot grow in an acid environment, only in an alkaline environment. So we must straighten out the pH in the body by bringing it into balance. Fungus cannot live in an oxidated only a non oxidated environment so are certain supplements to use to bring all these things into harmony.

Acidolphilus is an absolute must, restoring back this culture in the large intestines. There are 330 different cultures in the colon, 80 percent should be of the acidophilus nature. The 20 percent is generally made of indole, skatole, manila and candida. These are the bad things that cause problems. The acidophilus is destroyed by using birth control pills, antibiotics, cortisone and coffee.

These are other substances that are just as damaging. In order to bring the cellular structure back to the normal balance, we need to use vitamin C in the form of ascorbic acid and we need to use hydrcloric acid in the stomach as it is generally, greatly depleted. In fact, check for a hiatus hernia, as a majority of all people who have systemic candidiasis have a hiatus hernia, which restricts them from taking a deep breath and makes them unable to digest food.

We use caprylic acid, as it has the ability to kill fungus on contact. We use pau d'arco, as it also has the ability to kill fungus on contact and to protect the liver, which its number one job is to protect the bloodstream. The Lapacho tree from where pau d'arco comes from, grows in the rain forests of Brazil where the fungus grows abundantly, but you cannot find a single spore growing on a Lapacho tree. Garlic is also anti-fungal along with such herbs as black walnut, white oak bark, and red raspberry.

Diet needs to be emphasized as being super important. In fact, we have never seen anyone ever get well withoug a complete change of diet. The number one "Golden Rule of Health" states that we must stop putting poisons in the body and what poison is to one person may not be a poison to another. In fact, what is a poison to you now, probably may not be when you get your body chemically back into balance. We also have to change our environment when there is dampness, mold and fungus around us. We must either remove ouselves from the environment or remove the dampness, mold and fungus from the environment.

Laundry compounds should be changed to natural organic counpounds, getting away from the alkaline-based commercial soaps. We need to use an anti-bacterial, anti-fungicide in our laundry water so as not to pass this around to other members in the family and to continually re-infect ourselves. No one uses boiling hot water anymore and this is why this can happen. We need to change what we bath in, getting away from the alkaline-based soaps and using natural vegetable oil soaps that have a pH matching our skin so as not to destroy the invisible acid mantle that is on our skin. The acid mantle is there to protect us from something we catch, something that touches us, even something floating out of our air-conditioning ducts. Women should definitely not use tampons, as they will encourage fungal and bacterial activity such as toxic shock syndrome. One tip for the ladies: if they take a hot iron to the crotch area of their underclothing, this will help detroy fungal activity that is re-infecting them from their own clothing.

Alzheimers: Do not cook with aluminum foil as there is a heat transfer of aluminum to the food that you are cooking.

Amino Acids

All protein is composed of 22 amino acids. Amino acids are the building blocks of all protein of which there are 8 that are essential, in that the body can manufacture all 22 from these basic 8 amino acids.

Tryptophan	Phenylalanine
Leucine	Isoleucine
Lysine	Valine
Methionine	Threonine

They are called "essential" because they cannot be manufactured by the body themselves but must be supplied by foods in the diet.

If one essential amino acid is missing, or is present but in a low amount, protein synthesis in the body will fall to a very low level or stop altogether. If eating a protein food and one of the essential amino acids is in a much lower amount than the others, you will have what is called the limiting amino acid, and that is the factor determining the amount of body protein utilized by the body. For example, if a food contains 100 percent of a person's Valine requirement but only 20 percent of his Lysine requirement, it will result in only 20 percent of the protein in that food being used as protein by the body. The rest will be used as fuel rather than for replenishing of building tissue. Foods such as meat, poultry and dairy products are high in protein content and have a good proportion of essential amino acids. Many vegetables and fruits are low or missing some amino acids, thus rendering the amino acids present relatively useless.

This is one of the reasons why we should not try to live on a mono diet as the combining of foods can balance out our amino acid requirements. Eating a diet constantly deficient or lacking in amino acids can invariably cause rapid aging and disease in the body. Most cancer victims could benefit from the addition of amino acid supplements. The body's protein requirements can be easily met if the foods are properly combined in order to provide useable protein.

We need to emphasize the importance of balancing the amino acids to obtain the best possible protein from foods, Whereas the 8 essential amino acids cannot be manufactured, even in part by the combining of all the nonessential amino acids, the 8 amino acids can manufacture the other 14.

As we are learning more and more about amino acids, we are finding some very startling information. Researchers Durk Pearson and Sandy Shaw have found that a combination of amino acids when taken at bedtime, when the stomach is empty, will help you lose weight while you sleep. These amino acids safely stimulate the release of a growth hormone that boosts the rate at which your body burns fat and builds muscle. Because of increasing your rate of metabolism, you create more muscle and less fat. The growth hormone directs the body to burn fat at a rapid rate, and just as efficiently, build firm, taught muscle tissue.

This all-natural formation of amino acids is tryptophan, arginine, ornithine and lysine. Pearson and Shaw point out you could wake up pounds thinner and inches firmer without traditional dieting!

A proper balance of amino acids
- can enrich your bloodstream
- rejuvenate your skin
- build up your immune system
- regenerate your digestive system.

You need these life givers and life extenders in adequate supply in your daily food program. They hold the key not just to survival, but also to healthy self-rejuvenation.

Amino Acids have five functions:

1. They are building blocks used to make billions of body tissues and cells. These 'blocks' are the raw materials required to synthesize growth and repair in all parts of the body.
2. Thousands of enzymes needed for digestion of foods are created by amino acids. These wonder-workers also help produce hormones and glandualr secretions. Reproductive powers as well as virility and fertility depend upon a good amino acid supply.
3. Because of their structural properties, amino acids are vital for the functioning of the bloodstream.

4. Amino acids give you energy indirectly. A process takes place in the liver called deamination in which the liver converts an over-supply of amino acids of which 80 percent is converted. (56 percent into simple sugar (energy), 24 percent into waste (uric acid, urea) and 20 percent remains as amino acids and is left to circulate in the bloodstream. This is an extensive process and is unduly hard on the liver and kidneys.
5. Vital buffering agents for proper acid/alkaline balance.)

The 8 essential amino acids are:

1. L-Isoleucine
  •   Needed for hemoglobin formation
  •   Stabilizes and regulates the blood sugar and energy levels
  •   It is found in high concentration in muscle tissue

Deficiency: affects mental retardation and glycine production. It is needed for optimal growth in infants and nitrogen equilibrium in adults. A deficiency can lead to symptoms similar to those for hypoglycemia.

2. L-Leucine
  •   Is a stimulant to the upper brain, helping people to be more alert.
  •   Lowers elevated blood sugar levels.
  •   Promotes the healing of bones, skin and muscle tissue.
  •   Recommended supplement for those recovering from surgery.
  •   Must be taken in moderation, otherwise hypoglycemia may result.
  •   It is found in high concentration in muscle tissue

3. L-Lysine
  •   Improves concentration and mental alertness
  •   Utilizes fatty acids required in energy production
  •   Useful in the control and prevention of Herpes Simplex infection and cold sores
  •   It influences body growth, blood and circulation and

antibody formation.

- Needed for proper growth and bone development in children
- Helps calcium absorption and maintains nitrogen balance in adults.
- Aids in the production of hormones and enzymes.
- Helps in collagen formation and in the repair of tissue. Because it helps to build muscle protein, it is especially important for those recovering from surgery and sports injuries.
- Lowers high serum triglycerides
- It replaces the L-Lysine destroyed in food processing

Deficiency: Can cause "red spider webs" in the eyes as well as chronic fatigue, tiredness, loss of energy, inability to concentrate, irritability, hair loss, anemia, retarded growth, reproduction disorders.

L-Lysine's very important function is to assure adequate absorption of the mineral calcium. Another function of this amino acid is to form collagen. Without vitamin C or adequate protein to supply the amino acid Lysine, our wounds would not heal properly and we would become more susceptible to infections. One of the new discoveries for Lysine is in the treatment of herpes simplex. This viral infection is commonly known as cold sores or fever blisters. Herpes has become a major venereal disease in the United States and can cause serious complications in babies who may contact the disease from the mother during birth. Drs. Chris Karen and Tankersley, while working in the viral lab at the Cedars of Lebanon Hospital in Los Angeles, found that the amino acid Lysine inhibited it. They found that Lysine suppressed the symptoms of herpes in 96 percent of the 45 patients tested. Several patients were studied for as long as 3 years with complete remission of the herpes and no adverse reactions observed. Their report stated, "The pain disappeared abruptly overnight in virtually every instance, new vesicles (blisters) failed to appear, and resolution in the majority was considered to be more rapid than in their past experience." Inactive herpes can be controlled in most individuals with just one 500 mg. tablet of L-Lysine daily, but sometimes a larger dose is needed for the first few months, such as a 500 mg. tablet three times daily from 4 to 6 months. Treonine has been known to take on the role of a lipotropic to prevent fatty build-up in the liver.

4. L-Methionine
- Good source of sulphur
- Important in the treatment of rheumatic fever and toxemia resulting from pregnancy
- Used in the treatment of edema
- Used in the treatment of some cases of schizophrenia
- Research indicates a possible link to atherosclerosis and cholesterol deposits (assists in the breakdown of fats, preventing the build-up of fat in the liver and arteries, which obstructs blood flow to the brain, heart and kidneys.)
- Aids muscle weakness
- Helps to remove poisonous wastes from the liver
- Helps to regenerate the kidneys and the liver
- Influences hair follicles and hair growth (helps prevent brittle hair)
- Beneficial for allergic chemical sensitivities and osteoporosis
- Can be a natural anti-stress factor

Deficiency: Poor skin tone, hair loss, toxic waste build-up, malfunctioning of the liver

L-Methionine is a member of the lipotropic team which includes choline, inositol and betaine. Its function primarily, as a lipotropic, it is to prevent excessive fat in the liver. It increases the liver's production of lecithin and helps to prevent cholesterol buildup. It helps prevent disorders to the skin and nails. It also plays an important role as an anti-oxidant and free-radical deactivator.

All of these activities help to slow down the aging process. It gives the body the ability to chelate heavy metals and helps to eliminate the buildup of toxic minerals such as lead, mercury, and cadmium. It is also classified as an anti-fatigue agent.

5. L- Phenylalanine
- Controls hunger appetite suppressant due to release of cholecystokinin

- Improves memory, learning and alertness
- Produces neuro-transmitters that is used by the brain to manufacture norepinephrine
- Enhances sexual interest
- Helps alleviate depression, schizophrenia
- Because of its action in the central nervous system, it elevates moods.
- Should not be used by pregnant women or those with high blood pressure, PKU or with pre-existing pigmented melanoma.
- Precursor to tyrosine

Deficiency: Emotional upset, poor vascular health, some eye disorders, runaway appetite and weight gain

DL-Phenylalanine
- A non-addictive and non-toxic natural pain killer, especially arthritis
- Also is a very strong anti-depressant
- Increases mental alertness
- Suppresses the appetite
- Aids in Parkinson's disease

Phenylalanine—it has been claimed that learning may be improved with this amino acid and has proven to be an affective appetite depressant and diet aid. When Phenylalanine with the amino acid known as Aspartic Acid combines, it forms a new sweetener, aspartame. There is some questions, at this time, of brain damage in children when it is taken in large amounts. It is called Nutrasweet. If you have high blood pressure and are trying to lose weight with the aid of phenylalanine, don't forget to monitor your blood pressure.

Phenylalanine comes in two forms called D and L. L-(Laevo, or left-handed) phenylalanine is the form most commonly found in the high protein foods and is the form the body uses to make its own proteins. D-(dexto, or right-handed) phenylalanine is a nearly identical molecule to the L-form and is found in bacteria and plant tissue. The human body converts D-phenylalanine to L-phenylalanine before it is utilized in known bodily functions.

The role of dl-phenylalanine in the nutritional control of chronic pain-health professionals, pain treatment clinics, and scientific research papers have reported dramatic results in patients with severe, acute and chronic pain conditions including:

Migraine	Postoperative Pain
Neuralgia	Longstanding Whiplash
Joint Pain	Severe Premenstrual "Cramps"
Lower Back Pain	Rheumatoid Arthritis
Depression	Osteoarthritis

D- and DL phenylalanine (DLPA) work by intensifying and prolonging the body's own natural pain-killing response. Essentially, DLPA works because it inhibits endorphin degrading enzymes so that the endorphis produced by the brain last longer.

DLPA (DL-Phenylalanine) has been found to be 100 percent effective in the treatment of depression. Studies since show it to be particularly beneficial in cases of endogenous depression. This is the type of depression that is characterized by a decrease in energy and interest, feelings of worthlessness, and a pervasive sense of helplessness to control the course of one's life.

Significant improvement has also been achieved with people suffering reactive depression (thought to be caused by environmental influences such as death in the family) and involutional depression (an aging-related depression). DLPA has also been shown effective in manic depression, schizophrenic depression, and post-amphetamine depression.

6. Threonine
- Helps the digestive and intestinal tracts function more smoothly
- It also assists metabolism and assimilation
- Helps maintain protein balance in the body
- Important for the formation of collagen and elastin
- Helps to control epileptic seizures
- lipotropic agent (helps prevent fatty build-up in liver)

Deficiency: Indigestion, acid upset, stomach disorders, malabsorption, weak assimilation and general malnourishment

7. L-Tryptophan

- Anti-depressant
- Reduces anxiety, tension and promotes sleep, insomnia
- Lowers pain sensitivity
- Also aids in the control of alcoholism
- Necessary for production of niacin (produces nicotinic acid which may be useful in countering the effects of nicotine in cigarettes)
- Used by the brain to produce serotonin, a necessary neurotransmitter that transfers nerve impulses from one cell to another and is responsible for sleep
- Helps control hyperactive children, alleviates stress, is good for the heart, aids in weight control and enhances the releases of growth hormones necessary for the production of vitamin B-6
- Is used in the treatment of migraine headaches
- helps in reduction of blood fats for cholesterol

Deficiency: inability to sleep, poor skin coloring, brittle fingernails, prematurely aging skin, indigestion

As early as 1913 it was noted that a disease called pellagra was due to a deficiency of tryptophan. We know niacin to be the anti-pellagra vitamin and the body can manufacture niacin from dietary tryptophan. This amino acid has been used clinically as an antidepressant and has been used in PMS with good success. Women with PMS who had clinical signs of severe depression were found to have low levels of tryptophan.

Artery or heart spasms can occur in a human being and can cause a heart attack. This type of heart attack accounts for more than 15 percent of all heart deaths. L-Tryptophan supplements can conceivably reduce the risk of this type of heart attack.

L-Tryptophan has also been found to benefit those who have trouble sleeping. It has been found that in the research done in 1979 that L-Tryptophan when used as a sleep aid, it significantly decreased the time necessary to fall asleep. Dr. Ernest Hartman of Boston State Hospital and Tufts University School of Medicine has found that 1,000 milligrams (1 gram) of L-Tryptophan taken 20 minutes prior to going to bed reduces the time required to fall asleep by one-half. It also increased the duration of sleep, and improved the quality of sleep. You certainly don't have to take an "upper" the next day because you took a "downer" the night before.

L-Tryptophan does not work by drugging or depressing the central nervous system. L-Tryptophan returns normal function by merely making available for the body to use in making Serotonin. It does not seem to induce sleep during the day, but seems to be very effective at night as it must pass the blood-brain barrier. When taken singly at night, it can do so much more readily if there are no other amino acids trying to get through at the same time. L-Tryptophan and B complex are partners in the body.

The body will use some of the L-Tryptophan to make some of the B vitamin niacin (vitamin B-3) if a person is niacin deficient. Therefore, one may not get the full effect of the L-Tryptophan if one is not getting adequate niacin. One should consider taking a B complex with the L-Tryptophan. Dr. Federigo Sicuteri says it also may be effective in treating migraines. His research showed to be effective in about half of the migraine sufferers treated.

8. Valine
- Promotes mental vigor, muscle coordination and calm emotions
- It is used to treat severe amino acid deficiencies caused by addictions
- one of the amino acids found in high concentration in muscle tissue

Deficiency: Can lead to nervous ailments such as nail biting, sleeplessness, nervous reactions and generally poor mental health

OTHER AMINO ACIDS

L-Glutamine
- Used primarily as a brain fuel (improves intelligence)
- Alleviates fatigue and depression
- Used in the control of alcoholism
- Craving for sugar, mental ability, impotence, epilepsy,

senility, mental retardation and peptic ulcers
- Can readily pass the blood-brain barrier
- Used to protect against the poisonous effects of alcohol
- Has been used in the treatment of schizophrenia
- Used to treat ulcers and petit mal epilepsy

Older folks and others who are grouchy and cantankerous may become more cheerful.

L-Glutamic Acid
- 50 percent of the amino acid composition of the brain is represented by Glutamic acid
- Fuel for the brain
- It transports potassium across the blood-brain barrier
- It is used to treat epilepsy, hepatic coma, muscular dystrophy, mental retardation and insulin coma

L-Cysteine and L-Cystine work as antioxidants in the body and work closely with vitamin E and selenium. Each of these nutrients enhance the anti-oxidant role of the other. It has been used in the treatment of arthritis, both osteoarthritis and rheumatoid. It is necessary for the utilization of vitamin B6. L-Cystine protects against the damage from radiation by terminating the free radicals produced by radiation. It is also necessary to have adequate amounts to be able to excrete lead from the tissues. Because irreversible brain damage when allowed to accumulate. Durk Pearson and Sandy Shaw say that L-Cystine can "extend the life span, increase the growth rate of human hair, significantly decrease the health risk of smoking and drinking, stimulate the body's disease-fighting immune system, and block reactive hypoglycemia."

They caution that you should use three times as much vitamin C as Cystine. For example, if you take 1,000 mg. of Cystine you should take 3,000 mg. of vitamin C.

L-Cysteine
- Helps to minimize the random cross-linking by free radicals which can result in aged skin, hardening of the arteries, accumulation of age pigments, arthritis, cancer

- It is an effective antioxidant and scavenger of the free radicals
- It promotes healing from surgical operations and burns
- It stimulates white cell activity in the immune system for disease resistance
- It serves as a protectant at the cellular level agaisnt adverse effects of smoking and drinking
- It breaks down mucus in the respiratory tract
- It promotes the formation of carotene which is necessary for hair growth and maintenance
- It aids in iron absorption
- It is effective in preventing hangovers

Deficiency: Poor skin tone, hair loss, toxic waste build-up, malfunctioning of the liver

L-Cystine
- It stimulates white blood cell activity in the immune system necessary for disease resistance
- It is essential for the formation of the skin
- It promotes healing from surgical operations and burns

L-Tryosine has been found to play a role in controlling anxiety and depression. Dr. Alan J. Glenberg of the Department of Psychiatry of Harvard Medical School has found it will help in mental disorders. Dr. Glenberg reported considerable improvement in two patients whose longstanding depressions were not responsive to conventional drug therapy. An additional note on Tryosine, it is suggested that Tryptophan and Tryosine may be a better sleep aid than Tryptophan alone.

L-Tyrosine
- Appetite suppressant
- Fights fatigue and depression
- Helps cocaine addicts kick the habit—alleviates the withdrawal symptoms (depression, fatigue and irritability)
- Important in the treatment of anxiety, allergies and headaches

- Aids in the production of melanin (pigment of the skin and hair) and in the functions of the adrenal, thyroid and pituitary glands
- Growth hormone stimulant
- Considered an antioxidant
- Formed from phenylalanine

Histidine is necessary for the growth in children and is the amino acid from which a biochemical substance histamine is derived. Both histamine and histidine can chelate such trace elements such as copper and zinc. In some forms of arthritis, there is found an excess of copper and other heavy metals, so it is sometimes used for the treatment of arthritis.

L-Histidine

- Non-essential amino acid that has been found to be effective in the treatment of allergic diseases. Studies have shown that as the levels of dietary histidine increase, the concentration of histamine decreases. Histamine is a biochemical which occurs normally in the soft tissue of the body and is released during trauma and other stressful conditions
- It is also being investigated as a possible treatment for rhematoid arthritis ever since it was discovered that there appears to be less of it (about 1/4 as much) in the blood of arthritics as in the blood of non-arthritics
- Effective for cardiovascular diseases
- Abundant in hemoglobin
- Effective in treating allergic diseases
- Treatment of peptic ulcer
- Treatment of anemia
- Chelates to trace minerals copper and zinc
- Treatment of rheumatoid arthritis to remove heavy metals from tissues
- Important in production of red and white blood cells

Deficiency: Poor hearing or deafness, injuries to the nerve cells of the hearing mechanisms that make it difficult to distinguish words

L-Arginine
- Metabolizes body fat
- Tones muscle tissue
- Increases sperm count in males
- Aids in the healing of wounds
- Stimulates the immune system
- Blocks formation of tumors
- Causes the release of growth hormone
- Involved in liver regeneration
- Promotes the development of mature sperm
- Promotes detoxification of ammonia
- Helps in preventing premature aging

There is some evidence that two of the non-essential amino acids, histidine and arginine, cannot be made by the body fast enough to meet the requirements of young children, and so may be considered as essential for some individuals.

L-Carnitine
- Controls increases in body fat stores by converting nutrients into energy (is synthesized in the liver, purpose is to encourage fat metabolism in the muscles—that is, the utilization of fat as fuel for the generation of of energy.) This function is particularly important for the heart
- Enhances athletic performance
- Disperses excess calories (aids in weight loss)
- Decreases the risk for heart disease
- Vegetarians are more likely to be deficient in carnitine due to a diet that is low in lysine
- Enhances the effectiveness of antioxidant vitamins E and C.
- It is useful in the management of ischemic heart disease
- Plays an important part in the production of heat in brown fat
- It prevents the accumulation of ketones during weight loss
- It reduces blood triglycerides
- It increases the use of fat as an energy source

L-Glycine
- Used in the treatment of gastric hyperacidity, acidemia (acidity in blood)

- Used for low pituitary gland function
- For progressive muscular dystrophy
- Helps trigger the release of oxygen to the energy-requiring cell process
- It is the simplest amino acid
- It is an inhibitory neurotransmitter in the central nervous system
- It stimulates the release of growth hormone
- It is used as a food additive for a sweet taste
- Physiological functions (synthesis of hemin in hemoglobin)

L-Aspartic acid
- Improves stamina and endurance
- Increases resistance to fatigue
- Helps to protect the central nervous system
- Protects the liver by aiding in the removal of excess ammonia from the body.

It is involved in the transformation into other amino acids which are participants in glycolysis (the conversion of carbohydrates, glucose, etc., in cells), which takes place between protein amino acids and the citric acid cycle of cell oxidation and respiration. Through enzymatic action, the aspartic acid becomes pyruvic acid.

Scientific Advancements

GERMANIUM

This important trace mineral has been known of for over 30 years and its benefits have been well documented. But it was not allowed to be used in this country according to the FDA. As with most important health and medical facts, it takes many years to introduce them to the general public and to be accepted by the authorities in the individual field involved. So it is with germanium.

There is record of germanium being used in its inorganic form as early as 1922, when it was used by American doctors to treat anemia. However, a Japanese doctor, Dr. Kazuhiko Asai first synthesized the organic form as Ge-132 in 1967. This is the current organic form of germanium as is currently being used and studied with good or miraculous results.

Dr. Asai primarily worked with coal when he first became interested in germanium. Being a knowledgeable chemist, he knew that coal was rich in organic germanium so he developed the techniques for isolating it from the coal. He also made many human studies as to its healing benefits. He found that natural organic germanium was present in certain plants that are used extensively as healing herbs. These plants are ginseng, mushrooms, aloe vera, comfrey, garlic, shelf fungus and others. Germanium is also present in rich amounts in chlorella, wheat grass, barley greens, alfalfa, spiralina, blue green algae, and other chlorophyll rich products.

The results in the healing benefits of the organic germanium parallel the healing results of these chlorophyll healing substances. The advantage of using the germanium over the chlorophyll is that germanium is isolated and this isolated state, allows it to be used in a more concentrated way, thus yielding greater noticeable benefits of healing and maintenance in good health. This isolated concentration allows it to be individually tested to better ascertain its healing benefits and not wonder if other ingredients are responsible for any observed healing.

It can be understood that the trace mineral germanium's good to excellent results, are of its ability for the live cells to make better use of its available oxygen supple. Scientific observation and testing has produced the vital knowledge that all life is primarily dependent on an adequate supply of oxygen. Germanium has the proven ability to make the best possible use of oxygen and the ability to balance and render a much improved ability of the cells to utilize oxygen. This explains why germanium is useful and shows such good results in so many diseased conditions. Above and beyond even this in all the testing that has been done on germanium, it has never shown any adverse side effects. Thus far it has been proven to be nontoxic and yet, very powerful in its healing capabilities.

The thought has been presented that germanium has acted in the bloodstream as does hemoglobin and that this is the factor which is responsible for much of the increased healing benefits produced by its use. Dr. Asai in his work found that an intake of 100-300 milligrams of germanium a day improved most of the illnesses that he treated including:

- rheumatoid arthritis
- food allergies
- elevated cholesterol
- candidiasis
- chronic viral infections
- cancer and AIDS

Germanium has been shown to be a fast-acting pain killer when an intake of several grams has been given. Germanium works by attaching itself to molecules of oxygen, as does hemoglobin, which are carried by way of the bloodstream, into the body to improve cellular oxygenation. It is vital that the body receive oxygen to maintain immune system functioning ability. The increased supply of oxygen helps the body to rid itself of its toxins. Dr. Asai has the firm belief that prominent among cause of diseases is an insufficient oxygen supply to the bodies cellular systems. Research has shown that organic germanium is an effective way to increase tissue oxygenation due to its affinity for oxygen as is hemoglobin. Due to this ability, germanium has been beneficially used in the treatment of respiratory diseases including lung cancer.

Researchers have demonstrated that germanium exhibits a the ability to stimulate the immune system in cancer patients. It can be used to advantage in maintaining good health in healthy individuals. Germanium is known to normalize metabolic functions resulting in decreasing high blood pressure and cholesterol levels. The cumulative evidence suggests that germanium enhances the cell's ability to generate energy by raising the cell's oxygen supply. Since many disease symptoms are caused by the reduction of oxygen delivered to the cell level, it can well be understood that organic germanium will increase the over-all mental health and vitality.

The *Townsend Letter for Doctors* says, "Its oxygenation phenomenon allows greater organism function with reduced oxygen intake. It creates an oxygen economy with extremely fast-acting effects. Those with Raynaud's syndrome, for example, will feel warmth in the effected fingers and toes one-half hour after taking germanium. Healthy people will feel the warmth in a couple of minutes."

It is known that without oxygen, our cells and tissues begin to die within a few minutes. When one suffers a stroke, brain cells are destroyed because of clots and fatty deposits present along the lining of the arteries restricting blood flow containing vital oxygen. People who suffer a stroke may lose their ability to speak, write or read because some of the areas responsible for those functions have incurred brain tissue damage due to lack of sufficient oxygen. It would stand to reason that germanium might well constitute a prominent inclusion in any first aid pack as the cellular oxygen it would supple to effected nervous tissue could reduce any possible permanent brain and nervous damage.

Deficiencies in tissue's oxygen storage are, no doubt, the cause of most degenerative illnesses. Diseases are often characterized by hypoxia, an inadequate supply of oxygen to the cells and tissues. Researchers believe germanium provides the tissue cells with oxygen. There is a noticeable increase in the energy level when germanium is provided in sufficient quantities. Germanium's ability to increase tissue oxygenation well explains why it offers such valuable and measurable effects on maintaining healthy cells and organs.

Germanium's chemical structure helps nutritional supplements to bind or chelate (grab) toxic substances and remove them. Its chelating effect renders germanium especially helpful for mercury, cadmium and similar metal poisonings. Most all, people are subjected to mercury toxicity because of dental fillings, and to smokers in particular (smoking causes high cadmium toxicity). Due to its chelating ability, organic germanium functions as an antioxidant as well as an oxidant. Germanium helps to arrest osteoporosis by helping the body in restoring a normal calcium balance.

Germanium demonstrates it ability as an adaptogen, a nontoxic substance which normalizes body functions indirectly. Known adaptogens, such as vitamins C and E and Coenzyme Q10, improve one's capacity to cope with the increased pollutants of modern living such as air pollutants, electrical pollutants, freeway driving, television, computers and many others. Germanium is demonstrated to be beneficial by reducing cholesterol levels.

Germanium stimulates the body's natural defense mechanisms and is good for combating viruses, funguses and bacteria especially candida albicans, a yeast infection. Germanium does not directly kill viruses and bacteria, but increases the bodies' immune systems ability to do so. Germanium plays an active role in returning the body's defenses to normal so the body can rid itself of excess body toxins. Germanium is known to significantly enhance the body's production of interferon.

Cancer patients are immuno-deficient. Germanium aids cancer patients in restoring the body's defenses. A prime cause of cancer has been discovered to be oxygen deprivation in the cell. Research has observed that aerobic (oxygen-using) cells exhibit regular controlled growth patterns, anaerobic (oxygen-deprived) cells show abnormal growth. Germanium increases the supply of oxygen to oxygen poor tissue, such as cancerous growths and lessens the peroxidation of fatty acids. This has established germanium in the role of free radical pathology. Free radicals are highly reactive molecules which use up the oxygen supply, making it unavailable to the cells. When free radicals abound, tissue injury and disease states such as cancer can occur due to an insufficiency of oxygen in the cellular tissues.

There can be a remarkable prolongation in life spans with the availability and use of germanium. As we grow older, our systems accumulate an increase of free radicals. Free radical formation results in serious membrane damage that is responsible for age granules in cells. Some scientists believe that the body's ability to maintain a healthy immune system is vital in preventing premature aging and extending the quantity and quality of our lives. As people age, many experience a decline in their energy. Germanium may help to retain youthful vigor and a physical zest for life.

Germanium can act as a painkiller in painful conditions like rheumatoid arthritis. The ability of germanium to act as a pain killer is, no doubt, to be accredited to its ability to increase oxygen to the body and to the painful area in particular thus removing the cell oxygen deficit which is the cause of much of the painful rheumatic conditions. Germanium demonstrates remarkable analgesic effects which work in conjunction with its anti-tumor effects. It can reduce painful conditions and remove the need for excessive amounts of morphine. The increased oxygen available in the tissue saturated with germanium acts by increasing the activity of morphine at the receptor sites, and in addition, releasing self-made endorphins, germanium should be used only as organic sesquioxide.

- It acts as an anti-cancer agent, particularly where there is tumor metastasis, by activating macrophages and increasing production of killer cells

- A stimulus to interferon in the body for immune strength. Facilitates oxygen uptake, detoxifies and blocks free radicals
- Effective for viral/bacterial and fungal infections, osteoporosis, arthritis, heart, blood pressure and respiratory conditions. Success with leukemia, AIDS, brain, lung, pancreatic/lymphatic cancers

Herbal and Food Sources

Shelf fungus (Reishi and Shiitake mushrooms), garlic, ginseng, angelica, sanzukon, waternut, comfrey, boxthorn seed, wisteria knob, aloe vera, chlorella, pearl barley, tuna, oysters, green tea, onions, leafy greens.

CoQ10

Coenzyme Q10is a compound, the presence of which is required in order for an enzyme to function. Many of the B vitamins are coenzymes.

Coenzyme Q10 is a vitamin-like antioxidant that produces energy in heart cells and helps to normalize the pulse. Coenzyme Q10 was discovered in America in 1957, but was not then allowed on the market by the FDA. It has only been within the last 10 years that coenzyme Q10 has been commonly known and used in the United States. Since 1957, soon after its discovery, hundreds of university studies have confirmed that CoQ10 is essential for maintaining and supporting healthy immune and cardiovascular system functions.

Coenzyme Q10 is the nutrient that has the chemistry necessary to trigger the actual creation of cellular energy. CoQ10 is an integral part of the cell mitochondria, the subcellular components that are responsible for generating almost all of the total energy required by the human body, 95 percent. Organs such as the heart, liver, kidneys, spleen and pancreas, which require vast amounts of energy, must contain at all times high levels of CoQ10. University studies show that when levels of CoQ10 drop to 25 percent or lower of normal these organs cannot meet their energy requirements with major health problems resulting. In fact, if lower than 25 percent, death is just around the corner.

Further studies reveal that as we age we do not assimilate enough CoQ10 from the foods we eat, putting us on the brink of potentially serious health problems at all times. This accounts for the rapid way we can be overcome to illness for very quickly. We don't just catch something and die in a hurry. We spend years on the brink and finally we deprive the body one last time of the vital elements and compounds that we so desperately need.

CoQ10 promotes healthy gum tissue, is essential for heart valve integrity and supports metabolism, which is crucial for controlling and maintaining a healthy weight.

One of Parkinson's disease main symptoms is an involuntary shaking of the hands, the head or both. Coenzyme Q10 is one of the vital nutrients that are involved in the body's synthesis of acetylcholine and dopamine.

CoQ10 builds the immune fighting ability of your phagocytes and increases the efficiency of tissue detoxification. Coenzyme Q10 helps prevent heart disease, hypertension, diabetes, Alzheimer's disease and obesity and is helpful in their treatment. CoQ10 is an antioxidant which strengthen muscles, improving physical performance and endurance. It aids the body to adjust to higher altitudes and improves physical endurance. Coenzyme Q10 has shown excellent results in clinical use in periodontal disease, by speeding up healing time, stopping bleeding of the gums, reducing gum pockets and improving other factors associated with gum disease.

Clinical studies throughout the world have shown that CoQ10:

- aids in the prevention of toxicity from drugs used to treat many diseases associated with aging.
- energizes your body's cells supplying energy and endurance.
- nutritionally supports heart tissue; reduces the risk of heart attack (aids respiration of the heart muscle; provides a protective effect against viral-caused heart inflammations; helps prevent cardiac arrhythmias)
- Shares many of vitamin E's antioxidant properties.

Supplementation of Coenzyme Q10 may reduce angina episodes and improve cardiac function. Research has revealed that use of coenzyme Q10 benefits:

- Alzheimer's disease
- candidiasis
- diabetes
- may help in the prevention and control of cancer
- may help to heal duodenal ulcers
- mitral valve prolapse
- multiple sclerosis
- respiratory disease
- schizophrenia

CoQ10

1. Also used in the treatment of inflammatory gum disease.
2. Reduces high blood pressure without other medication.
3. Successful in combating angina and degenerative heart function.
4. Supplementation has a long history of effectiveness in boosting immunity, increasing cardiac strength, reversing high blood pressure, promoting natural weight loss, inhibiting aging and overcoming periodontal disease.
5. The body's ability to assimilate food source CoQ10 declines with age.
6. There are ten common Coenzyme Q's, but Coenzyme Q10 is the only one found in human tissue.

Sources

1. Found in rice bran, wheat germ, beans, nuts, fish and eggs
2. Mackerel, salmon, and sardines contain the largest amounts of Q1.

MERCURY-AMALGAM TOXICITY

The dangers of the silver-mercury-amalgam fillings has been known for over 100 years. The dentist is scared to death to admit the damage he has done sometimes knowingly, fearing you are going to come back and sue him for past problems. Model children have been turned into juvenile delinquents and many adults have suffered the problems that could not be diagnosed simply because of their fillings. As long as their fillings are in their mouth, they have a continuous absorption of the mercury poisons in their bodies. They have everything from tachycardia to an extremely slow heart beat to arthritis and even to allergies. They never seem to be able to be taken care of no matter what they do. The doctors have a big bucket that they throw multiple problems in and they call it Chronic Fatigue syndrome. These problems include Epstein-Barr virus, Candida albicans, in many cases cancer and others and these problems can never be taken care of until these fillings are removed.

Dr. Kupsinel states that, "Mercury vapor and organic mercury pass the placental barrier and may harm the fetus." Immediate responses to the point of remission have been seen in patients with Hodgkin's disease and leukemia once removal of the dental mercury fillings was done. Multiple sclerosis patients have thrown away their walkers after having the mercury amalgams removed.

There is an electro-galvanic test that can be used in order for the doctor to determine the sequential order of the mercury fillings to be removed in order to prevent a toxic flare-up of neurological symptoms. There have been studies for longer than 25 years proving that mercury is constantly being leached into the bloodstream via the saliva from the amalgam fillings. Deterioration of the jaw bone is noticed by bleeding of the gums and loosening of the teeth. Many times there is an identifying blue area in the gums near the tooth that is seen identifying mercury toxicity. This is referred to as a mercury tattoo and is a sign of mercury toxicity. One of the names given to this problem is Kawasaki's disease.

Following are some of the symptoms of mercury-amalgam toxicity:

- Depressed immune symptom
- Loss of self confidence
- Shyness
- Shortened attention span
- Fits of anger
- Insomnia
- Drowsiness
- Abdominal cramps
- Diarrhea
- Colitis
- Persistent cough

- Emphysema
- Shallow breathing
- Muscle weakness
- Fatigue
- Anemia
- Swelling or edema
- Loss of appetite
- Loss of weight
- Obesity (that does not respond to weight reduction programs

SHARK CARTILAGE

First the need, then the current facts studied, then an idea of what is needed to do the job. The job to be done was determined to be some way to slow down or retard, to as great a degree, as possible, new growth of blood vessels. The known facts were searched out and it was postulated that the substance needed was in cartilage, this was due to the *avascular* nature of cartilage. Bovine cartilage was first looked into, but it was determined that shark cartilage was where most of that product could be obtained. Shark cartilage had 1000 times more of the *avascular* substance than any other known source.

These facts were already known; research had been done on the subject and the research was then laid aside in files and left. By a fluke of circumstances, I. William Lane, as he states in his book, *Sharks Don't get Cancer,* stumbled over the information, discovered the research material and thanks to his previous education and job experiences (marine expert, nutritionist, and international businessman) he recognized the vital importance of the material. He was able to reinstate the research and assemble an interested and knowledgeable group to continue the investigation into the usefulness of sharks cartilage as having healing qualities. There was and is, understandably, opposition from the entrenched regulars in medicine and the pharmaceutical industry.

The work is being carried on successfully at the present time and a book has been written by Dr. I. William Lane which is a must to read on the subject of shark cartilage. The title of the book is *Sharks Don't Get Cancer.*

Though the following terms and their descriptions have been around since 1935 to the present time, these terms have not had a common usage, however due to the continuing influx of cancer and the search for the magic bullet to heal cancer and the tissue conditions in cancer and other healing conditions, these terms are and will continue to come increasingly into prominence. One such term is angiogenesi;, angio meaning "blood" and genesis meaning "formation of." So we are here referring to the formation of blood vessels, and the body making new blood vessels. Another word with the same meaning is "neovascularization" but it is not in as common a usage as that of "angiogenesis." It merely means the origin and development of blood vessels.

Angiogenesis describes the vascular building that takes place during ovulation and pregnancy. This same thing is happening in all wound healing and in any situation where there is need to restore or build tissue as all living tissue must be supplied, in an ongoing manner, with a continuing fresh supply of nutrients, always supplied by blood.

This process (angiogenesis) is only used by the body when there is injured tissue to rebuild, (promote healing) and in tumor formation. Cartilage has the characteristic of being very sparsely invested with blood vessels, less even than the denser portion of bones, as the physiology of cartilage does not require a rich blood supply.

It was postulated that the logical place to look for such natural inhibitors of angiogenesis (the formation of new blood vessels and/or capillaries), would be in tissue not requiring a rich blood supply (avascular in nature). The most common avascular tissue is cartilage. The thinking was, "cartilage is avascular, it contains vascular inhibitors of new growth." It had been discovered that shark cartilage contains, pound for pound, by far the most actively anti-angeogenetic substance known to man.

Dr. Robert Langer of the Massachusetts Institute of Technology and Dr. John Prudden, a Harvard trained physician, in their research have been able to extract and isolate a factor in cartilage that does inhibit tumor growth by reducing the formation of capillaries.

In 1976, Dr. Robert Langer showed that shark cartilage contained an inhibitor of new blood vessels in tumors. Dr. Judah Folkman of Harvard theorized that tumors could be completely prevented if the blood supply to any tumor could be controlled or lessened. We know that a blood supply is necessary for the sustenance of all life, so preventing the formation of a blood vascular formation in tumors could prevent tumor formation. In the search for a cancer cure in the conventional manner, some substance must be found that would prevent the formation of any tissue mass which is what a cancer formation is.

On the other hand, if you have abnormal growth of any kind, that growth must get its growth material from the blood. You need to stop this blood supply, how best to do this but to cut off this supply through diminishing its blood vessels. The blood vessels in tumors are fragile, immature and need replacing on an ongoing basis. Thus, reducing the ability to grow these vessels would slow down or stop the growth of the tumor or other growth tissue. The result would then be necrosis of the tumor, which would decay away. This has been observed when this tissue has been cut away, it is not pinkish but is gray bloodless tissue with the presence of air in the involved tissue, indicating the absence of blood.

Cancer is often considered a rapidly growing mass of tissue that is out of the control of the body. It is supposed that angiogenesis is an ongoing state kept in control by the anti-angiogenesis which the body produces and seems to have some control over.

So, we see that in the beginning of this research, there were several independent research physicians working on the belief that there was a possibility of isolating this anti-angiogenetic substance from a known source. That known source is being directed toward the shark. Sharks do not have bones as do most other fish. This has made them vulnerable even to the mild dolphins who are able, one on one, to kill sharks, so as to protect themselves or their young by butting the shark to death. This can happen because the shark has no bones to protect their inner organs. This is what makes the shark so important, in this case, as they have an abundance of cartilage from which to isolate and extract this anti-angiogenetic substance.

When scientists were curious as to why sharks didn't get cancer they asked the question, "What makes the difference?" The obvious fact came to their attention, sharks don't have bones. Next question was, so what? Now the investigation, and the subsequent answer. It takes vascularization to establish bone structure from cartilage that prevents the growth of blood vessels. There is! Can it be isolated and extracted? It can, and has been. Thus shark cartilage as an aid to mankind through the use of shark cartilage substance.

There are several discovered substances that have been found to be useful in the shark cartilage such as, 1) anti-angiogenetic substance, 2) ground pulverized shark cartilage mixed with other materials and sprayed over burned flesh and, 3) a host of other uses in degenerative diseases, like arthritis, inflammation of joints, enteritis effecting degeneration of the small blood vessels of the eye, psoriasis, a skin disease, and other uses some still undiscovered. The skeleton of sharks consists of pure cartilage, a hard gristly substance made up of proteins and complex carbohydrates.

In 1983, Dr. Anna Lee and Dr. Robert Langer finally isolated the "antiangiogenetic" substance, as theorized earlier, to exist. This factor was extracted from shark cartilage and has worked well to inhibit both blood vascular development and tumor formation. This inhibitor has proven to be 1,000 times more concentrated in shark cartilage than any other known source as opposed to bovine cartilage which depends on its ability to stimulate the immune system with mucopolysaccharides (complex carbohydrates) which has been positive, but not the significance in its ability to reduce capillary formation.

The end result when compared to the extract of shark cartilage is similar but actually coming from another direction. Complex carbohydrates from the bovine cartilage was the bovine factor that inhibited the formation of blood vessels. In the shark the actual single substance responsible for anti-angeogenesis has not been isolated and can not be identified. However, it is the more powerful of the two substances by far. Separately it was found that shark cartilage required less purification than bovine cartilage to achieve inhibition of angiogenesis. The obvious conclusion here is this newly discovered anti-angiogenetic factor should mostly do away with cancer.

If shark cartilage, as a treatment for cancer and other diseases is used successfully it would be well to improve on these results by combining with the shark treatment a natural cleansing program with vital nutrients such as vitamins, minerals, herbs, and fresh juices. There could be some possible problems with using this anti-angiogenesis substance without taking into consideration that cancer patients need physical support derived from improved nutrition. They need measures to properly cleanse and invigorate body toxin elimination.

In the Jules Bordet studies, 1,200 milligrams (1.2 grams) of dry cartilage per 1 kilogram (2.2 pounds) of body weight inhibited tumor growth. High daily doses of 50 to 60 grams are effectively given either as retention enemas or in part as enemas and in part orally.

Dr. I. William Lane and associates administered and recorded the resuilts of the Cuban Study. They were responsible for the organization of this study. Cuba supplied this team of researchers with a modern hospital facilities and the terminally ill cancer patients. It was reported to Dr. Lane's book "Sharks Don't get Cancer," that much improvement was noted and that there was rapid absorption of the substance when the treatment was first started.

Dr. Lane states, "The Cuban study is all the more remarkable when is it understood that all the patients under treatment were considered terminal and were in their last stages of life and that due to circumstances present in Cuba no vitamin or mineral supplementation was used in conjunction with the study program due to the absence of adequate nutrition available there, (malnutrition is common in Cuba at the present time.) Any future study of this magnitude will include a wide array of proven vitamin and mineral supplementations."

The shark cartilage was administered, either orally or rectally as a retention enema on the patients. A supportive program was not used but is vital to the success of any cancer healing program. However, substantial progress was noted with the administration of the shark cartilage. It was an informative venture which revealed many things of the methods of future administration of anti-angiogenesis substance.

It has been determined that the shark cartilage succeeded in stopping the tumor growth in the beginning by reducing substantially the growth of the capillaries that fed the metatastic tissue. There was encouragement that there has been a substantial breakthrough in the treatment of cancer as a result of the growth of cancer.

Many useful facts were gathered and important conclusions reached in the ongoing research conducted to date on shark cartilage. While shark cartilage extracts use in tumors and cancer are the focal points of general interest there are several other medical uses being investigated with different components of the cartilage.

Following are a few of the avenues being developed.
1. The shark cartilage extract with the anti-angiogenesis properties can be administered orally or rectally with equally good results.

2. There has been some question about stomach and intestinal irritation with bleeding when the extract from the shark cartilage was administered orally. This has been disproved.
3. High doses when taken orally has caused some very minor stomach irritation in some people, but this has not been serious. There has been no bleeding. When administrated rectally there has been only good results with no side effects (see following test results).
4. Shark cartilage, when administered rectally shows no gastric discomfort nor changes in the intestinal mucosa.
5. Shark cartilage extract has shown absolutely no toxicity at any dose level to date.
6. There has been positive pain relief in all cases where Shark Cartilage has been used. It has been thought that this pain reduction is the result of reduction in the tumor size.

Due to its anti-inflammatory and anti-antigenesis characteristics once shark cartilage is in a person's system it begins to work on a many different types of diseases. Among these diseases are arthritis, psoriasis, and enteritis. These diseases have already shown healing response to shark cartilage. Also benefits have been demonstrated, on diabetic retinopathy, neovascular glaucoma, and macular degeneration, these have been discussed in scientific journals. These are age old diseases that have been around for a while. It is thought that, if this shark cartilage holds up to its expectations there could be a drop in these diseases as a positive side effect to its use, especially with the increased age expectation on the rise.

Rheumatoid arthritis often exhibits an abnormal inflammatory condition that host an abnormal capillary increase which can destroy the joint cartilage and can cause calcification. Persistent angiogenesis is apparently the basic cause of the disease. The same problem is involved with osteoarthritis which is a destructive disease of the articular cartilage of the joint. In many of the diseases discussed it is well to add the question, "What comes first the disease condition to be treated or wrong life practices that need to be corrected." It has a obvious answer, but most treatment is based on a treatment for the disease condition not on a correction of its real cause. In a severe manifestation of the degenerative disease both the treatment of the disease and a change of the life style cause should be instituted by the doctor or the health professional or the self treating patient.

One of the outstanding features of shark cartilage is that in the treatment of degenerative diseases it is nontoxic, inert, making it safe to use in cooperation with other forms of treatment. It is considered that the shark cartilage's healing action is its ability to retard the growth of blood vessels and its stimulation of the immune system, thus it does not interfere with other forms of therapy or medication, whether complex, drastic or simple in nature.

Another condition that shark cartilage has been successful in helping is Psoriasis recognized by an increased production and peeling of the skin with the visible reddening under the surface of the skin, denoting a rich supply of capillaries in the outer layers of the skin with a thickening of the skin above this reddened area. When the shark cartilage was administered subcutaneously, total remission was experienced with the skin becoming smooth again but the reddening remaining. With continued shark cartilage therapy the capillary network, causing the reddening, shut down and normal skin appearance returned.

Shark cartilage when used with skin grafts for burn victims was very useful in preventing rejection of the grafts by the body. This is at present a routine procedure.

The use of shark cartilage is a breakthrough in medical treatment of many untreatable diseases to date. Time will bring forth many more uses of shark cartilage in the treatment of the ill.

Shark cartilage products now on the market contain not only the pure source of mucopolysaccharides but also is combined with Reishi mushroom, a powerful immune stimulating agent, which has a long history of use in China and which can be very effective in restoring health.

Common sense needs to be practiced in administrating the anti angiogenesis shark cartilage.

1.   A patient with known heart damage, where the heart needs rebuilding, it should be obvious that, such a patient should not take an angiogenesis inhibitor, which is a product that will slow down, suppress, and stop normal angiogenesis. The heart muscles needs nutrients via the blood vascular system, for rebuilding purposes.

2.   Another person who should avoid this medication is a pregnant women that is in the act of building a family, and a women who wants to get pregnant. A pregnant woman who is building a blood

network to feed the developing embryo should not use shark cartilage. Women who are attempting to conceive should also avoid taking shark cartilage which may interfere with vascularization during the menstrual cycle. Any condition where there is need to build healing tissue.

3. People with deep surgery and who need new blood vessels to speed healing, should not take shark cartilage, nor should people involved in a major muscle-building program.

4. Children's blood vessels are still developing, so a careful consideration should be given regarding their use of angiogenesis inhibitors.

This turns out to be a part of the age old battle between the medical doctors and the irregulars, the "minutemen" and "minutewomen" of the present age. We are battling for the rights to use those drugless healing agents, of which shark cartilage is a chink in the armor of useful products, from being removed by the drug industry.

Raw Glandular Concentrates
(Protomorphagens)

In large measure, aging is a function of the health of the glands. If the glands are youthful and if old weak cells are replaced by new strong ones, then the body itself is young. You are only as old as your glands!

When we use raw glandulars, we are using the organ tissue to provide the nutrients that our own organs must have in order to replenish themselves. We use specific glandulars for specific parts of the body, such as brain would supply the proteins, enzymes, vitamins, and other nutritional elements needed to replace brain cells. Adrenal helps the adrenal; liver, liver, etc.

When a pack of wolves kills a deer, or a pride of lions pulls down a zebra, the first parts of the prey they eat are the organs, such as kidney, adrenals, pancreas, thymus, heart, liver, etc. Primitive human hunters followed the same pattern. They ate the organs first and would save the meat for later. They were then assured of getting the best and most concentrated nutrition. In prehistoric times when humans were hunters, a diet rich in organ meat guaranteed them necessary nutrition. Even when people settled to the cities, organs remained a very important culinary item. This was also true in the United States until the end of the 19th century, when organs began losing ground to red meat.

The major increase of muscle meat in our diets has been one of the major causes of arthritis and other degenerative diseases, because this type of meat is acid producing. Raw glandulars come from livestock. After the animals have been slaughtered, the organs are removed under carefully controlled conditions and made into the final product which is called a glandular concentrate. It is also called "raw" because it contains all the biological material found in the original tissue which could be destroyed through heat. Europeans have pioneered the therapeutical use of glandular materials. Dr. Paul Niehass, the dean of Europe's glandular therapists, injected finely ground fresh gland tissue into patients suffering from such diseases as diabetes, premature aging and sexual disfunction. In over 12,000 injections he reported one clinical success after another, sometimes even actually restoring function to glands that had practically ceased to work.

Glandular concentrates have been used in successful treatments for such things as hypoglycemia, prostate cancer and kidney stones. You don't have to wait for disease to strike in order to enjoy the advantages of raw glandulars, nor do you have to endure the pain or expense of cell injections. Laboratory studies using radioactive tagging indicate that the vital factors in glandular material leave the intestines intact and travel through the body through the lymph system. This guarantees that the raw glandular concentrates taken by mouth does deliver effective nutrition to the glands.

Physicians have for years been injecting liver extracts, expecting, and most of the time receiving, admiral results in many disorders. Some would like to attribute these effects from the iron and the B-complex factors inherent in liver, but when the same quantities of these substances are used alone, the results are not the same.

It is believed that glandular tissue concentrates in some way transmit specific DNA stimulants. DNA (Deoxyribonucleic Acid) is the master chemical blueprint for building of new cells, and the RNA (Ribonucleic Acid) is the messenger chemical that carries out the DNA's instruction. Life continues normally until the DNA ceases to form the RNA after which cell regeneration is seriously inhibited or stopped. When this becomes widespread, death is the final result.

In the 1977 issue of the *Journal of the International Academy of Preventative Medicine*, Dr. Ivan Popov gives two important reasons of supplementing the diet with raw glandular concentrates. They are poor nutrition and aging. That pretty much means all of us, as no one escapes aging, especially now when organ meats are rarely included in the diet, glandular nutrition affects almost everyone.

Raw glandulars include a wide variety:

adrenal	kidney
pituitary	thymus
stomach	thyroid
pancreas	duodenum

male testes and prostate   female ovaries and uterus
brain   heart
liver

If you feel that you are in need of a glandular, you should at least consider a multiglandular concentrate. Such a product contains tissue from all the principal glands and helps provide balanced nutrition for these important organs. Multiglandulars can be taken regularly with complete safety, just like supplemental vitamins and minerals. Your multiglandulars are usually a low potency and will just support those important glands, not try to take them over such as drugs do in the body. When taking singular glandular concentrates, they shouldn't be taken on a regular basis for any longer than 9 to 12 weeks, as they have a tendency to take over the job the gland should be doing.

Tests conducted in both Europe and the U.S. indicate that freeze-drying yields the most biological active raw gland concentrates. Freeze-drying preserves all gland functions. Raw glandulars should be made only from animals that have been grazed solely on clean range land. Look for freeze-dried concentrates from imported livestock. Remember—you are only as old as your glands, nourish those important organs well and you will enjoy the youthful glow of good health for years and years to come. The key concept in glandular therapy is that like cells help like cells.

Appendix

TABLE 1*

Some Nutrients Dependent on Each Other

*Supplied through the courtesy of the Nutrionics Literature Search, 624 N. Victory Blvd., Burbank, CA 91502 (213) 841-7200.

Nutrient	Complementary Nutrients	Anti-Vitamins	Bodily Functions Affected	Deficiency Symptoms
Vitamin A Fat Soluble	B complex, choline, C, D, E, F, calcium, zinc	alcohol, coffee, cortisone, excessive iron, mineral oil,	body tissue reparation and maintenance (resist infection). Visual purple production (necessary for	allergies, appetite loss, blemishes, dry hair, fatigue, itching burning eyes, loss of smell, night blindness,
rough		vitamin D	night vision.)	dry skin, sinus trouble, soft tooth enamel, susceptibility to infections
Vitamin B1 Water Soluble	B complex, B2, folic acid, niacin, C, E, manganese, sulphur	alcohol, coffee, fever, raw clams, sugar (excess), stress, surgery, tobacco	appetite, blood building, carbohydrate metabolism, circulation, digestion (hydrochloric acid production), energy, growth, learning capacity, muscle tone maintenance (intestines, stomach, heart)	appetite loss, digestive disturbances, fatigue irritability, nervousness, numbness of hands & feet, pain & noise sensitivity, pains around heart, shortness of breath

TABLE 1 Continued

Nutrient	Complementary Nutrients	Anti-Vitamins	Bodily Functions Affected	Deficiency Symptoms
Vitamin B2 Water Soluble	B complex, B6, niacin, C, phosphorus	alcohol, coffee, sugar (excess), tobacco	antibody & red blood cell formation, cell respiration, metabolism (carbohydrate, fat, protein)	cataracts, corner of mouth cracks & sores, dizziness, itching burning eyes, poor digestion, retarded growth, red sore tongue
Vitamin B6 Water Soluble	B complex, B1, B2, pantothenic acid, C, magnesium, potassium, linoleic acid, sodium	alcohol, birth control pills, coffee, radiation (exposure), tobacco	antibody formation, digestion (hydrochloric acid production), fat & protein utilization (weight control), maintains sodium potassium balance (nerves)	acne, anemia, arthritis, convulsions in babies, depression, dizziness, hair loss, irritability, learning disabilities, weakness
Vitamin B12, Water Soluble	B complex, B6, choline, inositol, C, potassium, sodium	alcohol, coffee, laxatives, tobacco	appetite, blood cell formation, cell longevity, healthy nervous system, metabolism (carbohydrate, fat, protein)	general weakness nervousness, pernicious anemia, walking and speaking difficulties

Nutrient	Complementary Nutrients	Anti-Vitamins	Bodily Functions Affected	Deficiency Symptoms
Biotin, B complex Water Soluble	B complex, B12, folic acid, pantothenic acid, C, sulphur	alcohol, coffee, raw egg white (avidin)	cell growth, fatty acid production, metabolism (carbohydrate, fat, protein), vitamin B utilization	
Vitamin C Water Soluble	all vitamins & minerals, bioflavonoids, calcium, magnesium	antibiotics, aspirin, cortisone, high fever, stress, tobacco	bone & tooth formation, collagen production, digestion, iodine, conservation, healing (burns & wounds), red blood cell formation (hemorrhaging prevention), shock & infection resistance (colds), vitamin protection (oxidation)	anemia, bleeding gums, capillary wall ruptures, bruise easily, dental cavities, low infection resistance (colds), nose bleeds, poor digestion
Vitamin D & Fat Soluble	A, choline, C, F, calcium, phosphorus	mineral oil	calcium & phosphorus metabolism (bone formation), heart action, nervous system maintenance, normal blood clotting, skin respiration	burning sensation (mouth throat), diarrhea, insomnia, myopia, nervousness, poor metabolism, softening bones & teeth

TABLE 1 Continued

Nutrient	Complementary Nutrients	Anti-Vitamins	Bodily Functions Affected	Deficiency Symptoms
Vitamin E Fat Soluble	A, B complex, B1, inositol, C, F, manganese, selenium, phosphorus	birth control pills, chlorine, mineral oil, rancid fat & oil	aging retardation, anti-clotting factor, blood cholesterol reduction, blood flow to heart, capillary wall strengthening, fertility, male potency, lung protection (anti-pollution), muscle and nerve maintenance	dry, dull, or falling hair; enlarged prostate gland; gastrointestinal disease; heart disease; impotency; miscarriages; muscular wasting; sterility
Vitamin F Unsaturated eczema, fatty acids	A, C, D, E, phosphorus	radiation, x-rays	artery hardening prevention, blood coagulation, blood pressure normalizer, cholesterol destroyer, glandular activity, growth vital organ respiration	acne, allergies, diarrhea, dry skin, dry brittle hair, gallstones, nail problems, underweight, varicose veins

Nutrient	Complementary Nutrients	Anti-Vitamins	Bodily Functions Affected	Deficiency Symptoms
Choline Water Soluble	A, B complex, B12, folic acid, inositol, linoleic acid	alcohol, coffee, sugar (excessive)	lecithin formation, liver & gallbladder regulation, metabolism (fats, cholesterol), nerve transmission	bleeding stomach ulcers, growth problems, heart trouble, high blood pressure, impaired liver & kidney functions, intolerance to fats
Folic Acid Water Soluble	B complex, B12, biotin, pantothenic acid, C	alcohol, coffee, stress, tobacco	appetite, body growth & reproduction, hydrochloric acid production, protein, metabolism, red blood cell formation	anemia, digestive disturbances, graying hair, growth problems
Inositol	B complex, B12, B2, C, Phosphorus	alcohol, coffee	artery hardening retardation, cholesterol reduction, hair growth, lecithin formation, metabolism (fat & cholesterol)	cholesterol (high), constipation, eczema, eye abnormalities, hair loss

TABLE 1 Continued

Nutrient	Complementary Nutrients	Anti-Vitamins	Bodily Functions Affected	Deficiency Symptoms
Niacin Water halitosis, Soluble	B complex, B1, B2, C,	alcohol, antibiotics,	circulation, cholesterol level reduction, growth,	appetite loss, canker sores, depression, fatigue,
	phosphorus	coffee, corn, sugar, starches (excessive)	hydrochloric acid production, metabolism (protein, fat, carbohydrate), sex hormone production	headaches, indigestion, insomnia, muscular weakness, nausea, nervous disorders, skin eruptions
Pantothenic Acid Water Soluble	B complex, B6, B12, biotin, folic acid, C	alcohol, coffee	antibody formation, carbohydrate, fat, protein conversion (energy), growth stimulation, vitamin utilization	diarrhea, duodenal ulcers, eczema, hypoglycemia, intestinal disorders, kidney trouble, loss of hair, muscle cramps, premature aging, respiratory infections, restlessness, nerve problems, sore feet, vomiting
PABA, Para Amino-benzoic Acid B complex	B complex, folic acid, C	alcohol, coffee, sulfa drugs	blood cell formation, graying hair (color restoration), intestinal bacteria activity, protein metabolism	constipation, depression, digestive disorders, fatigue, gray hair, headaches, irritability

Nutrient	Complementary Nutrients	Anti-Vitamins	Bodily Functions Affected	Deficiency Symptoms
Calcium	A, C, D, F, iron, magnesium, manganese, phosphorus	lack of exercise, stress (excessive)	bone & tooth formation, blood clotting, heart rhythm, nerve tranquilization, nerve transmission, muscle growth & contraction	heart palpitations, insomnia, nervousness, muscle cramps, arm & leg numbness, tooth decay
Chromium	none	none	blood sugar level, glucose metabolism (energy)	atherosclerosis, glucose intolerance in diabetics
Copper	cobalt, iron, zinc	zinc (high intakes)	bone formation, hair & skin color, healing processes of body, hemoglobin & red blood cell formation	general weakness, impaired respiration, skin sores
Iodine	none	none	energy production, metabolism (excess fat), physical & mental development	cold hands & feet, dry hair, irritability, nervousness, obesity

TABLE 1 Continued

Nutrient	Complementary Nutrients	Anti-Vitamins	Bodily Functions Affected	Deficiency Symptoms
Iron	B12, folic acid, C, calcium, cobalt,	coffee, excess phosphorus, tea,	hemoglobin production, stress & disease resistance	breathing difficulties, brittle nails, iron deficiency
anemia	copper, phosphorus	zinc (excessive intake)		(pale skin, fatigue), constipation
Magnesium	B6, C, D, calcium, phosphorus	none	acid alkaline balance, blood sugar metabolism (energy), metabolism (calcium & vitamin C)	confusion, disorientation, easily aroused anger, nervousness, rapid pulse, tremors
Manganese	none	calcium, phosphorus (excessive intake)	enzyme activation, reproduction & growth, sex hormone production, tissue respiration, vitamin B1 metabolism, vitamin E utilization	ataxia (muscle coordination failure), dizziness, ear noises, loss of hearing

Nutrient	Complementary Nutrients	Anti-Vitamins	Bodily Functions Affected	Deficiency Symptoms
Potassium	B6, sodium	alcohol, coffee, cortisone, diuretics, laxatives, salt (excess), sugar (excess), stress	heartbeat, rapid growth, muscle contraction, nerve tranquilization	acne, continuous thirst, dry skin, constipation, general weakness, insomnia, muscle damage, nervousness, slow irregular heartbeat, weak reflexes

Table 2
Recommended Optimum Personal Allowances (OPAs) for Vitamins

	Weight (±20 lbs.)	Height (±5')	Fat-Soluble Vitamins			Water-Soluble Vitamins (Essential)									Water-Soluble Vitamins (Contested)			
			Vitamin A (IU)	Vitamin D (IU)	Vitamin E (IU)	Vitamin C (mg)	Folic Acid (mcg)	Thiamin B1 (mg)	Riboflavin B2 (mg)	Niacin B3 (mg)	Vitamin B6 (mg)	Vitamin B12 (mcg)	Biotin (mcg)	Pantothenic Acid (mg)	Inositol (mg)	PABA (mg)	Pangamate (mg)	Bioflavonoids (mg)
MALES																		
Age: 19-35	147	69																
Lower limit			5,000	400	100	1,000	500	50	50	100	50	50	50	100	100	50	25	50
Upper limit			10,000	600	200	2,000	1,000	150	150	300	150	150	150	200	200	150	75	100
Age: 36-50	154	69																
Lower limit			5,000	400	200	1,000	500	100	100	100	100	100	100	100	100	100	25	50
Upper limit			10,000	600	400	3,000	1,000	150	150	300	150	150	150	200	200	150	75	100
Age: 51+	154	69																
Lower limit			10,000	400	400	2,000	500	100	100	200	100	100	100	100	100	100	25	50
Upper limit			15,000	600	600	4,000	1,000	200	200	400	200	200	200	300	300	200	50	100
FEMALES																		
Age: 19-35	128	65																
Lower limit			5,000	400	100	1,000	500	50	50	100	100	50	50	100	100	50	25	50
Upper limit			10,000	600	200	2,000	1,000	150	150	300	200	150	150	200	200	150	75	100
Age: 36-50	128	65																
Lower limit			7,000	400	100	1,000	500	100	100	100	200	100	100	100	100	100	25	50
Upper limit			12,000	600	300	3,000	1,000	150	150	300	300	150	150	200	200	150	75	100
Age: 51+	128	65																
Lower limit			10,000	600	400	2,000	500	100	100	200	100	100	100	100	100	100	25	50
Upper limit			15,000	800	600	4,000	1,000	200	200	400	200	200	200	300	300	200	50	100

NOTE: IU = International Unites; mg = milligrams; mcg = micrograms

TABLE 3

ANALGESIA IN HUMAN PAIN PATIENTS IN RESPONSE TO D-PHENYLALANINE

Condition	Duration	Prior Treatment	Time on DPA	Result
Whiplash	2 years	Empirin, Valium	3 days	Complete relief, 1 month
Osteoarthritis, fingers, thumbs of both hands	5 years	Empirin, aspirin	maintained	Excellent relief; joint stiffness reduced
Rheumatoid arthritis (left knee), osteoarthritis of hands	several years	Empirin & Codeine	1 week	Considerable relief
Low back pain, neck pain	several years	90 acupunctures	3 days	Low back pain gone; walked one mile
Low back pain	several years	Spinal fusion, percutaneous nerve stimulation	3 days	Much less pain
Low back pain	several years	Laminectomies, Depomedrol, percutaneous nerve stimulation	3 days	Good to excellent relief
Fibrositis of muscle	?	Empirin	3 days	Pain gone, recurred after 2 days
Migraine headache	several years		2 days	Good relief, may prevent recurrence
Cervical osteoarthritis plus postoperative pain	?	?	2 days	Very little pain
Severe lower back pain	several years	Empirin, Valium	3 days	Excellent relief

Alzheimer's Disease

Completely eliminate the use of all aluminum cooking utensils and aluminum drinking utensils.

Stop the use of aluminum foil, especially in baking as then is a transfer of aluminum to the food through heat. Even the use of aluminum foil when baking a fowl or roast also allows the transfer of aluminum through heat—*this also includes baked potatoes and pies!* The use of a Muscle Response Test will quickly show the fallacy of using aluminum foil in cooking.

Exercise regularly.

Use glandulars to restore the RNA and the DNA factor *(refer to the section of glandulars)*, and multiple glandulars would probably be best. Do not use antiperspirant deodorants as they contain aluminum chlorohydrates. Also commercial baking powder contains aluminum.

* Oral chelation is a method of taking orally into the body those substances that will break down and help to remove such detrimental things as calcium, lead, mercury, aluminum, and, other substances that cause harm to the brain and can cause hardening of the arteries (arteriosclerosis). You are only as healthy as your circulatory system in that its job is to provide every cell in the body with adequate amounts of nutrition, and when it slows down, the cells begin to starve and then we become candidates for strokes and heart attacks. The A.M.A. feels the only answer is by-pass surgery—we feel there are others.

ALZHEIMER'S DISEASE

- Avoid aluminum cookware, aluminum deodorants, soft drinks and fruit juices in cans
- Stay away from alcohol
- Stay away from food additives, antacids, shampoos that have aluminum in them.
- Alzheimer's: Do not cook with aluminum foil as there is a heat transfer of aluminum to the food that you are cooking

SEE AILMENT SECTION IN THIS BOOK

CANDIDA ALBICANS

Candida Albicans is a friendly bacteria in the bowel. As long as it is in the bowel, there is no problem. It is when it causes fungus infection outside of the bowel that problems begin to show up.

Candida Albicans can cause thrush and vaginal infections. It can, in fact, mimic almost any disease from eye infection to allergy to colitis, cystitis, gastritis, brain tumor, multiple sclerosis, and even insanity. There are even more symptoms: depression; lethargy; agitation; loss of memory and concentration; headaches; dizziness; insomnia; disturbance in smell, taste, vision, hearing; sensitivity to chemical odors, fragrances, foods; weight loss or gain; hay fever; bronchitis; hives, menstrual irregularities; bloating; diarrhea or constipation; Crohn's disease; arthritis; myasthenia gravis; vaginal yeast infections; and prostatitis. It is also believed that the majority of all prostatitis is Candida Albicans.

Major problems come from the use of Cortisone, birth control pills, and antibiotics. Many allergies are caused by the hidden candida fungi. People who have developed susceptibility to this problem must follow a very strict diet in order to bring the ever present Candida under control. Certainly improving the immune system and restoring it to its natural state is the best advice that can be given.

The medical profession uses a drug called Nystatin—it is an anti-fungi drug. There are also many herbs that are anti-fungal.

Candida is often misdiagnosed. Another one is Premenstrual Syndrome. Candida Albicans and Premenstrual Syndrome go together like twin sisters. Symptoms of the two conditions are quite similar and should be treated concurrently for a complete cure. Premenstrual Syndrome, they have found, is majorly involved with the pituitary and thyroid glands, which influence the hormone balance in women.

The use of acidophilus is a must as it is one thing that will contain and control the Candida in the colon. It has been through the loss of the acidophilus bacteria that the Candida was allowed to escape from the bowel, causing its problems.

There are many things that will destroy the acidophilus in the colon such as red meat, which is generally high in antibiotics that are given to the animal in order to guarantee that it will make its way to the slaughterhouse. Coffee also destroys the acidophilus bacteria.

Although we need to stay away from milk products, acidophilus (though made from milk) is not a problem. Generally 10 fifty-million acidophilus capsules twice a day will get the job done if used for approximately three months. The person is sometimes a year to two years bringing the Candida completely under control and destroying it at the cellular level.

Multiple applications of acidophilus taken over a 24 hour period is absolutley necessary to restore acidolphilus culture in the colon. The best time to take acidolphilus is before bed time, first thing in the morning or as far away from food as possible.

DIETARY SUPPRESSION OF CANDIDA ALBICANS

The yeast grows on sugar and starch and is fed by gluten containing grains. Gluten grains include wheat, oats, rye, and barley.

Do not eat sugar or sweets. This includes products made with honey or molasses as well as sugar.

Do not eat wheat, oats, rye, or barley. Corn, rice, potatoes, buckwheat, and millet may be eaten in very small quantities by most individuals. *Some people, however, must temporarily exclude all of these starchy foods from the diet.* Milk (even raw) encourages Candida growth. Avoid milk and milk products except butter.

Yeast, molds, and fungi cross-react. When taken in food or even breathed in high concentrations, they trigger symptoms and diminish the body's resistance to Candida. Bathrooms and air vents should be kept clean and dry. Yeast, mold and fungus should he minimized in foods. Yeast is used in food preparation and flavoring: Commercial breads, rolls, coffee cakes, pastries, etc. Beer, wine, and all alcoholic beverages. Most commercial soups, barbecue potato chips, and dry roasted nuts.

Vinegar and vinegar-containing foods such as pickled vegetables, sauerkraut, relishes, green olives, and salad dressing. Lemon juice with oil may be used as a salad dressing. Soy sauce, cider and natural root beer.

Yeast is the basis for many vitamin and mineral preparations. Tryptophan is often derived from yeast. Molds build up on foods while drying, smoking, curing and fermenting. Avoid pickled, smoked, or dried meats, fish, and poultry, including sausages, salami, hot dogs, pickled tongue, corned beef, pastrami, smoked sardines and other fish that have been dried or smoked.

Bacon should be avoided. Country-style cured pork, of all kinds is loaded with mold.

Dried fruits such as prunes, raisins, dates, figs, citrus peels, candied cherries, currants, peaches, apples, and apricots should be avoided. All cheeses (including cottage cheese), sour cream, buttermilk, and milk should be avoided. Chocolate, honey, maple syrup and nuts accumulate mold and should not be eaten. Melons (especially cantaloupe) and the skins of fleshy vegetables or fruits accumulate mold during growth. Avoid canned or frozen citrus, grape, and tomato juice. Avoid all canned or frozen foods which contain citric acid. Mushrooms are fungi. Do note eat them. Drinking coffee destroys Acidophilus in the colon, releasing the Candida and enabling it to get into the bloodstream. Eating fruit will boost blood sugar levels and encourage yeast growth. Fruits and fruit juices must be temporarily omitted from the diet.

Teas, including herb teas, and spices are dried foods and accumulate molds. Avoid some herb teas and dried spices.

We need to emphasize that any vitamin supplements taken should be yeast-free until the Candida is under control, then you can return to your normal supplements with yeast in them.

What is Left to Eat?

PROTEINS:

Fish, chicken, turkey, duck, seafood, eggs, pheasant, quail, lamb, veal. In other words, animals if the meat is fresh instead of dried, smoked, pickled, or cured.

VEGETABLES:

All vegetables are potentially acceptable. Only starchy ones such as potatoes and sweet potatoes must be avoided by some people.

Is it Possible to Eat Out?

Yes! *Just order carefully.* Skip the cocktail. Have oil and lemon juice on your salad. Order meat, chicken, or other animal protein that is prepared without sauces which might contain *sugar, mushrooms, wheat as a thickener, and other harmful ingredients. Broiled or plain items are obvious, the safest choice. Steamed vegetables are perfect!* **Skip bread, crackers, and dessert.**

The use of such herbs as Garlic, Red Raspberry, Pau D'Arco, Sarsaparilla, Sage, White Oak Bark, and Black Walnut are all recommended as they are antifungal herbs *(refer to **The Little Herb Encyclopedia, Revised** for more information on these herbs)*. Certainly the use of Vitamin A, which is the antibiotic vitamin, will enhance the immune system—that along with Vitamin C. Some physicians are recommending as high as 200,000 i.u.'s of Vitamin A a day. The use of acidophilus is a *must!*.

One good naturopathic physician has found that we should be on a diet not to exceed 80 grams of carbohydrates a day.

ADDITIONAL RECOMMENDATIONS

- Check for a Hiatus Hernia
- Acidophilus - on an empty stomach
- Caprylic acid
- Pau d'Arco tea (bulk) - 1 quart a day
- Garlic
- Stop using antibiotics, steroids, oral contraceptives, all drugs
- Do colon cleansing
- Change what you bathe in as well as what you wash your clothes in
- Change the yeast environment
- Wear cotton clothes (underwear etc.) Use a germicide for clothing.
- Good hygiene, bathing frequently is important, using pads instead of tampons because they encourage fungal activity

SEE AILMENT SECTION IN THIS BOOK

MULTIPLE SCLEROSIS AND ALS

AVOID:

Eggs	Fried Foods
Wheat	Corn
Rye-Oats	Cucumber
Chocolate	Onions
Spinach	Radishes
Mild	Tomatoes
Sodas	Olives
Cocoa	Peanut Butter
Coffee	Pickles
Nuts	Relishes
Strawberries	Spices
Dry Fruits	Tobacco Smoking
Prune Juice	Gluten
Pork	Yeast
Fish	Bananas
Red meat	Avocados
Shell fish	Novacaine
Cheese	

USE:

B-Complex (yeast-free)
B12 (yeast-free)
Vitamin E
Vitamin C
Lecithin
Calcium & Magnesium
Substituted Polyunsaturates
Fats for saturated ones
*Evening Primrose Oil

Multiple Male Glandular or Multiple Female Glandular
Cod Liver Oil - 5 grams
Vegetable Oil - 10-15 grams
Oral Chelation
Mineral Maintenance
Vitamin A & D
Histamine
Curane
Exercise - Energizer
Reverse Osmosis (R.O.) Water
*Scullcap
*Combination 8
*HVS
*REX

ADDITIONAL RECOMMENDATIONS FOR MULTIPLE SCLEROSIS & ALS

- Avoid animal fat
- Increase consumption of essential fatty acids (EFA₂s)
- Increase cholesterol intake as the myelin sheath that disappears in Multiple Sclerosis is made almost exclusively of cholesterol.
- Remove mercury fillings
- Eat green vegetables and juices

SEE AILMENT SECTION IN THIS BOOK

References:
Dr. Boines
Delare Med. Journal Vol. 40
#2 February, 1968, p. 34

Dr. Jonez

*Refer to *The Little Herb Encyclopedia, Revised* by this author for further information on these herbs.

PREMENSTRUAL SYNDROME
(PMS)

Premenstrual Syndrome has just recently come to light as it was passed off for many years by the medical profession who claimed it was just women wanting attention when in actuality it is a body completely out of balance screaming for help. (Refer to Candida Albicans).

The use of a multiple glandular would be very beneficial. Also the need for Vitamin E is a must. Such herbs as Black Cohosh and Dong Quai need to be considered. Refer to The Little Herb Encyclopedia Vol. II for further information on the use of herbs in this condition.

ADDITIONAL RECOMMENDATIONS

- Stay away from salt, caffeine, sugar in any form, red meats, alcohol, processed foods, junk foods or fast foods and do not smoke.
- Check for Hiatus Hernia
- Eat plenty of fresh vegetables

SEE AILMENT SECTION IN THIS BOOK

Bibliography

Adams, Ruth. *The Complete Home Guide to All the Vitamins.* New York: Larchmont Books, 1972.

Adams, Ruth, and Murrah, Frank. *Minerals: Kill or Cure.* New York: Larchmont Books, 1976.

Barnard, Julian, *Bach Flower Remedies.* Hilman Printer, Frome, Somerset, Great Brittian 1979 pgs 52.

Battista, Al, *Candida Albicans.*

Bieri, John G. "Fat-soluble vitamins in the eight revision of the Recommended Dietary Allowances." *Journal of the American Dietetic Association 64* (February 1974).

Bland, Jeffrey Ph.D., *The Key To The Power Of Vitamin C and Its Metabolites.* keats Publishing Company, New Canaan, Connecticut, 1989, pgs 31.

Bliznakov, Emile M.D., *The Miracle Nutrient CoEnzymeQ10.* Bantum Books, 1986, pgs 16.

Borsaak, Henry. *Vitamins: What They Are and How They Can Benefit You.* New York: Pyramid Books, 1971.

Bullock, Shelia, *Homeopathy, What is it?* Naturally Yours, Dallas, 1992, 29.

Burke, Arnold W. Jr. *Inositol.* Hawkes Publishing, Inc., Salt Lake City, Utah 1982 pg. 26.

"Candida Albicans." Maureen Salaman Interviews Al Battista, N.D., *Health Express,* November, 1984.

Chaitow, Leon, D.O., *Amino Acids in Therapy.* Healing Arts Press, Rochester, Vermont, 1988, pg. 112.

Chancellor, Philip M. *M.D. Dr. Philip M. Chancellor's Handbook of the Bach Flower Remedies.* Keats Publishing, Inc. New Canaan, Connecticut, 242.

Clinkard, C.E. M.B.E., *The Uses of Juices.* C.E. Clinkard, 1960, pgs 32.

Eades, Mary Dan M.D., *The Doctor's Complete Guide to Vitamins and Minerals.* Dell Publishing Co., New York, NY, 1994 pgs 511.

Ebon, Martin. *Which Vitamins Do You Need?* New York: Bantam, 1974.

Erasmus, Udo, *Fats and Oils.* Alive Books, Vancouver, British Columbia, Canada, 1986 pgs 356.

Erdmann, Robert Ph.D., with Jones, Meirion, *The Amino Revolution.* Simon and Schuster, New York, NY, 1987 pgs 248.

Goodhart, Robert S., and Shills, Maurice E. *Modern Nutrition in Health and*

Disease. 5th Ed. Philadelphia: Lea and Febiger, 1973.

Grace, David, B.S., D.C. and Maryonen, Karen, M.F.S., *The Missing Element Organic Germanium.* American Institute of Health and Nutrition, 1989, pgs. 14.

Gregory, Scott J., O.M.D., *A Holistic Protocol for The Immune System.* Tree of Life Publications, Joshua Tree, CA 1989, pgs. 88.

Griffen, LaDean. *Please Doctor, I'd Rather Do It Myself . . . with Vitamins & Minerals.* Salt Lake City: Hawkes Publishing, Inc., 1979.

Hoffer, Abram M.D., Ph.D., *Vitamin B3 (Niacin) Update.* Keats Publishing Company, New Canaan, Connecticut, 1990 pgs 31.

Horne, Steven, *Sharks-Man's Best Friend/ or Invite a Shark to Dinner.* Nature's Field Volume 9 No. 1, January/February 1993, Springville, UT, 1993, pgs. 23.

Kamen, Betty, Ph.D., *Germanium: "A New Approach To Immunity".* Nutrition Encounter, Inc., Larkspur, CA, 1987, pgs. 35.

Kiminski, Patricia, and Katz, Richard, *Flower Essence Respertory Flower Essence Society,* Nevada City, CA, 1986 pgs 192.

Kaslof, Leslie, The Bach Remedies, A Self-Help Guide, Keatas Publishing Co., New Canaan, Conn.

Katz, Marcella. *Vitamins, Food, and Your Health.* Public Affairs Committee, 1971, 1975.

Kupsinel, Roy B. M.D., *A Patient's Guide to Mercury-Amalgam Toxicity.* Pub. By Roy B. Kupsinel, M.D., Oviede, ? pgs. 23.

Lane, I. William, Dr. and Comac, Linda, *Sharks Don't Get Cancer.* Avery Publishing Group, Inc., Garden City Park, NY, 1992, pgs. 192.

Lec, William II. R.PH., Ph.D., *Amazing Amino Acids.* Keats Publishing Co., 1984, pgs. 16.

Lieberman, Shari and Bruning, Nancy, *The Real Vitamin & Mineral Book.* Avery Publishing Group, Inc. 1992.

Martin, Marvin. *Great Vitamin Mystery.* Rosemont, IL: National Dairy Council, 1978.

McCraw-Hill Book Co. New York city, *Nutritional Almanac.* 1979.

Miller, Bruce B. Dr., *Beta-Carotene.* Institute for Preventive Health Care, Fort Worth, TX, 1985 pgs 28.

Mindell, Earl. *Earl Mindell's Vitamin Bible.* New York: Rawson, Wade Publishers, Inc., 1980.

Mondale, Earl, *Earl Mindless Vitamin Bible,* Rawson, Wade Publishers, Inc.,

New York, NY, 1980.

Null, Gary and Steve. *The Complete Book of Nutrition.* New York: Dell, 1972.

Passwater, Richard A. Ph.D., *Beta-Carotene.* Keats Publishing Company, New Canaan, Connecticut, 1984 pgs 26.

Passwater, Richard A. Ph.D., *Cancer Prevention and Nutritional Therapies.* Keats Publishing Co., New Canaan, Connecticut, 1978 pgs 230.

Passwater, Richard A. Ph.D., *Vitamin E Updated.* Keats Publishing Company, 1983 pgs 26.

Pfeiffer, Carl M.D., Ph.D., *Mental and Elemental Nutrients.*

Rodale, J.I., *The Complete Book of Minerals for Health.* 4th ed. Emmaus, PA: Rodale Books, 1976.

Rosenberg, Harold, and Feldzaman, A.N. *Doctor's Book of Vitamin Therapy: Megavitamins for Health.* New York: Putnam's, 1974.

Sehnert, Keith W. M.D., *The Garden Within.* Health World Magazine Burlingame, CA, 1989, pgs. 32.

Smith, Lendon H., M.D., *The Complete Home Health Advisor.* Woodland Health Books, Pleasant Grove, Utah, 1994 pgs 380.

Somer, Elizabeth, M.A., R.D., *The Essential Guide to Vitamins and Minerals.* Harper Collins Publishers, 1992, pgs. 403.

Ulene, Art M.D. and Ulene, Val M.D., *The Vitamin Strategy.* Ulysses Press; Berkeley, CA, 1994 pgs. 279.

"Vitamin-Mineral Safety, Toxicity and Misuse." *Journal of the American Dietetic Association,* 1978.

Wade, Carlson, *Amino Acids Book,* Keale Publishing Co., New Cannan, CN, pgs. 145.

Wade, Carlson. *Magic Minerals.* West Nyack, NY: Parker Publishing Co., 1967.

Wallach, J.D. DVM, ND, and Ma Lan, MD. MS, *Let's Play Doctor!.* Wholistic Publications, Rosarito Beach, Baja-California, Mexico, pgs. 200.

Webster, David, *Acidophilus & Colon Health,* Nutri-Books, Denver, CO, 1980, pgs. 24.

Werbach, Melvyn R., M.D., *Nutritional Influences On Illness.* Keats Publishing Company, 1987 pgs 504.

Yiamouyiammis, John Dr., *Flouride the Aging Factor.* Health Action Press, 1986, pgs. 204.

Index